Praise For Sleep, Interrupted

"There are many good books on better breathing. But none of them address why you need to breathe well when sleeping. Let Dr. Steven Park, an ENT physician, show you how you can breathe better while sleeping. Not only will this improve your energy, it can also save your life."
— CHRISTIANE NORTHRUP, M.D., AUTHOR OF NEW YORK TIMES BESTSELLER, *THE WISDOM OF MENOPAUSE*

"So many health problems result from sleep interrupted by breathing problems, poor sleep position, and other causes, yet few physicians make the connection and treat accordingly. This book will begin to change that and lead people to better health."
— ERIC BRAVERMAN, M.D., AUTHOR OF BESTSELLER, *YOUNGER YOU*

"Dr. Park's revelation of the vicious cycle of interrupted sleep and health problems turns the medical community on its head. More importantly, it provides answers for so many who struggle to understand why they feel so lousy, and how they can feel better."
— JACOB TEITELBAUM, M.D., LEADING AUTHORITY ON CHRONIC FATIGUE SYNDROME, AUTHOR OF BESTSELLER, *FROM FATIGUED TO FANTASTIC*

"Sleep Interrupted" is a seminal manuscript which not only reviews the upper airway anatomy and physiology in a concise reader-friendly fashion, but more importantly postulates associations between poor sleep and some everyday maladies in a manner heretofore unaccomplished. This is must reading for anyone who sleeps or breathes."
— STEPHEN LUND, M.D., CO-DIRECTOR, SLEEP DISORDERS INSTITUTE, NEW YORK CITY

"Many physicians treat only the symptoms of illness. Dr. Park carefully identifies what is causing millions of us to be sick, and shows us how to get and stay healthy and happy."
— JAMES, O'KEEFE, M.D., AUTHOR OF *THE FOREVER YOUNG DIET AND LIFESTYLE*

"The concepts in this book hold so much promise for a Kuhnian paradigm shift in the knowledge and practice of conventional medicine."
— DOROTHY HUNG, PH.D., ASSISTANT PROFESSOR, DEPARTMENT OF SOCIOMEDICAL SCIENCES, MAILMAN SCHOOL OF PUBIC HEALTH, COLUMBIA UNIVERSITY

"This is an excellent book that covers sleep and the consequences of not receiving good restorative sleep in an inviting, conversational style. Once you read this book, you'll know more about sleep-breathing problems than most doctors. It's a must read for anyone with chronic sleep or fatigue issues, and especially for all healthcare practitioners."
— **BRIAN PALMER, D.D.S.**, SLEEP APNEA RESEARCHER AND BREASTFEEDING ADVOCATE

"Billions of dollars are spent every year in intensive care units throughout the United States, attempting to treat and salvage patients at the end stage of chronic conditions. In contrast, very little time and effort is invested, in the education of the lay public, in recognizing and treating sleep disorders that can lead to a number of these chronic conditions. This outstanding and simply written book does just that. A must read."
— **ANITA BHOLA, M.D.**, FCCP, ATTENDING PHYSICIAN, CRITICAL CARE MEDICINE, SLEEP, PULMONARY AND CRITICAL CARE MEDICINE, ASSISTANT PROFESSOR, ALBERT EINSTEIN COLLEGE OF MEDICINE

Sleep, Interrupted:

A physician reveals the #1 reason why so many of us are sick and tired

Sleep, Interrupted: A physician reveals the #1 reason why so many of us are sick and tired

For information about this title or to order other books and/or electronic media, contact the publisher:

Jodev Press, LLC
330 West 58th Street, Suite 610
New York, NY 10019
www.jodevpress.com
866-693-9558

Library of Congress Control Number: 2008931401

ISBN: 978-0-9802367-0-5

Printed in the United States of America

Book and Cover design by: 1106 Design

To my patients

Sleep, Interrupted:

A physician reveals the #1 reason why so many of us are sick and tired

Steven Y. Park, M.D.

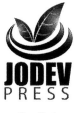

JODEV
PRESS

New York

Table of Contents

Section 3: Modern Day Solutions For Your Sleep-Breathing Problem

Acknowledgements

WRITING THIS BOOK has been a journey. This may be a common phenomenon for many first time authors, but each author's journey is uniquely different with personal significance. The entire process of writing and publishing this book has changed my life for the better. When I first conceived of the idea for this book, it was a daunting thought: taking time not only to write the book, but coordinating and organizing the entire team involved in the process, on top of running a surgical practice, being a husband and father of two boys. However, something strange happened—on top of finishing and publishing the book in about a year, I've enhanced my relationship with my wife, Kathy, rediscovered the joy of running, and have a new sense of purpose in what I do and why I do it.

John Eggen and everyone at Mission Marketing Mentors were instrumental in laying the groundwork for the systematic and time-tested methods that I used to write and publish this book. John, you are truly a master at what you do, and you definitely live out your mission of spreading your learned wisdom to eager students in your program. I also wish to thank the coaches (Lorna McLeod, Kim Olver, and Leslie Malin) that have helped to keep me grounded throughout the year. To my accountability partners, Bruce Hoffman and George Wissing, thanks for keeping me accountable.

Thanks to Beth McHugh, my editor down under, for her skill and patience. Graham Van Dixhorn, you are truly a whiz at creating dazzling cover copy. Thanks also go to the team at 1106 Design for their excellent work on the cover and interior design. An acknowledgment also goes to Jill Gregory for her skill and mastery in creating the illustrations for this book.

To all the book and chapter reviewers—this book is infinitely better because of your thoughtful input and constructive comments. Despite your busy schedules and overwhelming demands, you found time to read my manuscripts and to provide practical and sometimes critical suggestions: Dr. Christiane Northrup, Dr. Dean Ornish, Mary Shomon, Dr. James O'Keefe, Dr. Jacob Teitelbaum, Dr. Brian Palmer, Dr. David Buchholz, Dr. Anita Bhola, Dr. Dorothy Hung, Dr. Melanie Herrold-Smith, and Dr. Kasey Li. Thank you Dr. Bernie Seigel for your inspiring comments on inspiration.

Thanks also goes to all the people that I bugged repeatedly with title testing: Mike O'Neil, Juan and Kate Franco, Dr. George Alexiades, Dr. Boosara Goldin, Dr. Seth Dailey, Grace Marin, Deborah Lynch, Michelle Lee, Dr. Yelena Averbukh, Dr. Peter Hung, Rita Lombardi, Jay Easterling, and Dustee Hullinger.

I'm also grateful to all my patients for trusting me enough to reveal the critical elements that ultimately consolidated into the sleep-breathing paradigm. I can't think of a greater sense of professional satisfaction than connecting with and understanding what each of you are telling me beyond the obvious.

Finally, I am most grateful to my wife Kathy, who supported me through my ups and downs, emotional and financial roller-coasters, who was absolutely instrumental in the development of this important message that this book tries to convey.

List of Acronyms

Every effort was made to describe fully every acronym used in this book when first presented. However, here are the full descriptions of some of the more commonly used acronyms for your convenience.

ADHD	attention deficit hyperactivity disorder
AHI	apnea hypopnea index
Apgar score	simple reliable method to quickly assess the health of a newborn child immediately after birth
BMI	body mass index (calculate by dividing weight in pounds by height in inches squared and multiplying by a conversion factor of 703; or kg/m^2)
CFS	chronic fatigue syndrome
CPAP	continuous positive airway pressure
CRP	c-reactive protein
ENT	ear nose throat
GERD	gastroesophageal reflux disease
HMS	hyoid myotomy with suspension
IBS	irritable bowel syndrome
LPRD	laryngopharyngeal reflux disease
MMA	maxillo-mandibular advancement
MOGA	mandibular osteotomy with genioglossus advancement
OSA	obstructive sleep apnea
REM	rapid eye movement
TMJ	temporo-mandibular joint disease
TSH	thyroid stimulating hormone
UARS	upper airway resistance syndrome
UPPP	uvulopalatopharyngoplasty

Preface

The significant problems we face cannot be solved at the same level of thinking we were at when we created them.

— **Albert Einstein**

"I used to be on top of the world."

This is a quote from a former business executive whose slowly deteriorating job performance coincided with severe fatigue, lack of focus and poor concentration.

A woman in her thirties is frustrated about the fact that a few years ago, she was the top-performing employee in her company but now can barely carry out her job due to progressive and intense fatigue during the day.

Another young woman reports that her life is falling apart, and has recently started taking antidepressants. Her job performance is suffering as well, and she's spending too much time consulting too many doctors.

These three patients all came to see me initially for recurrent sinus infections and constant nasal congestion. It's common knowledge in medicine that people with chronic infections are usually tired and don't sleep well. The pain, infection, fever, and other aspects of chronic disease keep the patient up at night, leading to poor sleep quality and lack of energy during the day.

Over the past few years, I have seen countless patients in similar situations, and I used to think that their career and life situations were independent of their current medical problems. Now I realize that I was dead wrong.

I slowly began to see a link. All three of the above patients, as well as countless others who consulted me, had one thing in common. And it was quite simple. None of them were getting a good night's sleep.

You could argue at this point that maybe job stress and poor performance could lead to poor sleep, and in particular, insomnia. But all these patients had another common feature, which is the fact that they all preferred not to sleep on their backs. This is what turned the current disease paradigm upside-down for me.

If this were a problem purely due to sleep issues only, then there would be no need for this book. But there's one more piece of the puzzle that completes the picture. And this is the fact that all the patients I was seeing also had some kind of breathing problem, which was worse at night, especially in certain sleep positions. My hunch was eventually confirmed when definitive treatment for these sleep-breathing problems led to dramatic improvements, not only in how patients felt during the day, but also with their various other medical problems as well.

Sleeping and breathing are things that we all take for granted. When your nose is stuffy during the day, you will feel uncomfortable, and take measures to breathe better. Similarly, sleep is something we don't consciously think about when we're sleeping, and when we don't sleep well, we'll be wondering how we can sleep better the next day. No one ever realizes that they did not sleep well because they were not breathing well. This connection is never made. But these two events are intrinsically related, and when I first saw how profound an impact poor breathing has on sleep, it opened up a whole new world for me. It radically changed the way I practiced medicine and surgery, and later led me to the development of the sleep-breathing paradigm, which I describe in this book.

A paradigm is defined as a worldview underlying the theories and methodology of a particular scientific subject. What I'm proposing in this book was described by one of my colleagues as a kind of paradigm "shift." It doesn't disprove or discredit conventional, orthodox medical teachings, but presents how we may look at "worldviews" from a completely different perspective. I will refer to the concepts presented in this book as my "sleep-breathing paradigm."

Some of my good-meaning colleagues and reviewers remarked that the concepts may seem too complicated and that I need to somehow make it simpler, bringing it down to a fifth grade reading level. I decided not to take that advice, as doing so would be a disservice to my readers, who deserve an intelligent, lucid and logical explanation for their unexplained health problems. Instead, I decided to write in a conversational tone, as if I'm talking with you face to face during a consultation.

This sleep-breathing paradigm actually poses an interesting dilemma. Evolutionary biologists have long observed that the beneficial aspects of speech acquisition and language have also been accompanied by an unexpected negative side effect: only humans can choke and die. This is due to the unique oral anatomy we possess that allows us the power of communication. I will add to this another proposed side effect—that due to various degrees of inefficient breathing while sleeping, a number of common medical and mental health disorders can arise as a result.

If you think about it, breathing is the most fundamental physiologic activity that we all must do to survive. Breathing nourishes our bodies with oxygen, as well as removing carbon dioxide. Breathing also has other life-promoting implications, as in the phrase, "the breath of life." If there is an impediment to breathing of any kind, then it is logical that life and well-being can be interrupted, leading to various ailments and illnesses.

This new paradigm is not meant to be a definitive treatise on health and disease. Think of the concepts presented in this book not as an alternative or even a contradiction of current medical thinking, but as an added dimension in a multi-dimensional model. What started out as a simple mental exercise in my mind ended up being more than just a theory. It blossomed into a unique and useful tool by which many chronic medical conditions, as well as various ear, nose and throat conditions, can be explained and treated. In the coming chapters, you'll read how I came to realize this paradigm, along with all the supporting clinical experiences and published research studies that helped to solidify the process.

An amazing realization that came to me early on was the fact that, for the most part, the paradigm never contradicts any existing accepted clinical models. It agrees with or reconciles often contradictory views on a given subject. It's also exciting to constantly discover new clinical studies on various health issues that reinforce my paradigm—strengthening connections between known co-existing conditions, but more importantly, forging new links between medical conditions that were previously considered unrelated.

Some of you may be thinking by now that this book may be about obstructive sleep apnea. Yes, I do cover this condition, but it is only a small portion of my sleep-breathing paradigm. Obstructive sleep apnea is a distinct clinical condition which is at the extreme end of the picture that I am describing, and although not the main focus of this book, you will find more practical information about it here than many other books devoted entirely to it, including medical textbooks. Looking through the lens of the sleep-breathing paradigm will also change the way you think about obstructive sleep apnea.

Unfortunately, the group of people who most need to read and understand this book will be very resistant to it. I'm talking about other physicians. They will dismiss the findings in this book as being purely anecdotal, and not based on rigorously controlled large-scale research studies. But when was the last time a "definitive" prospective, large-scale, randomized, placebo-controlled, double-blind research study changed the way doctors practice medicine? When it comes to old habits, doctors can be the most stubborn old dogs of this world. Medical students are taught that they should look at the patient as a whole, but later in practice, it's much more glamorous looking for a magic bullet to cure cancer or an infection—if we can only find that one gene or molecule that leads to a particular cancer or depression. I can't tell you how often I come across medical articles in *The New York Times* that describe the discovery of a new technique or a new gene, where at the end of the article, states something to the effect that this exciting discovery could potentially lead to a cure in the future. How often does this ever happen?

Knowing what we know about sleep-breathing problems and health issues, it's shameful how little physicians in general ask (really ask) about the quality of the patient's sleep. All too often, a sleeping pill is prescribed without getting to the root cause of the problem.

Borrowing from the "can't see the forest for the trees" analogy, imagine that all the individual leaves of a tree represent all possible diseases that are known in humans. If you see the tree from above, all you see is a massive bunch of leaves. But if you look at it from below, you see that the main trunk connects to a number of thick branches, which divide further into smaller branches, and so on, until the smaller branches lead to all the leaves. In a similar way, inefficient breathing due to partial or total obstruction at night has been shown scientifically to directly or indirectly cause not only high blood pressure, but various other medical ailments described in coming chapters.

It seems to me that most research these days is focused on the extreme end process of an illness. Scientists today look for better ways of fighting bacteria after an infection begins, but almost never search for what can be done to prevent the infection from taking hold in the first place. The same applies to heart disease. The Western health model is centered around: "What can we do to prevent inflammation and damage *after* a heart attack?" instead of "What can we do to *prevent* heart disease from happening in the first place?" Treatment after a heart attack is important, but as long as you know that there are good ways of treating the effects of a heart attack, you may not be inclined to do very much in your earlier years to prevent the heart attack from even happening. You may comment at this point that doctors are already doing this by giving cholesterol lowering pills and anti-hypertensive medications. What I propose is the possibility that there will be no need at all for blood pressure or cholesterol medications if ineffective breathing patterns were corrected.

I will also allude to an observation that research in the fields of cardiovascular and cancer medicine seems to be working in parallel, but independently, almost like two parallel tree branches side by side. The real breakthroughs will happen when someone notices the common branch that divides into the two respective smaller branches. I'm not in any way implying that my sleep-breathing paradigm is the main trunk of the tree; rather, I see it as a larger tree branch from which many more illness and disease stem.

We physician-scientists are still heavily influenced by stereo-typical concepts of health and disease. Most physicians still believe that disease is an invasive, detrimental process that happens to a healthy, disease-free individual. One of the reasons that alternative and complementary medical fields are booming these days is that they provide an alternate explanation about what health and disease is. Some of these fields stress that it's not so much what's attacking your body, but how your body responds to the attack that's important. This preventive model is ideal. There are other systems or programs that tout anything as being curative, as long as it's not from the pharmaceutical industry. Undoubtedly, many of these treatments work, while many others don't. The problem is that you can't know whether or not it works until you try it. Some people end up taking a shotgun approach and try everything.

If you're reading this book, I'm assuming that you are interested in taking responsibility for your own health, and are open to new ideas and possibilities. Be warned: Some of my suggestions and hypotheses in the coming chapters will be controversial, perhaps even heretic. I just ask that you keep an open mind and try to see common conditions such as depression, high blood pressure or menopause through the viewpoint of the proposed sleep-breathing paradigm.

My hope is that this paradigm stimulates enough interest so that open-mind physicians can take these concepts and use it to the benefit of their own patients. If you are suffering from any of the various ailments described in this book, then this book may shed new light on why you feel the way you do. Every few weeks, I have a patient in my office that breaks down in tears once they finally understand for the first time why they are suffering, going from doctor to doctor, frustrated by all the unsuccessful treatments and confusing infor-mation. I don't expect that the concepts presented in this book will revolutionize the world, but my aim is to encourage people to do what the old Apple Computer commercials said: "Think Different." In this age of relativity, we must be willing to think differently about why we become ill, rather than what to do after we become ill. But once you are successful at thinking differently, you must then take action to see any benefits. Different chapters will elicit different reactions from different people.

The first part of this book describes how I came to discover my paradigm, some basic anatomy relevant to the paradigm, and other clinical concepts that will form foundations for later chapters. The middle section describes various common medical conditions from the viewpoint of the sleep-breathing paradigm. Finally, the concluding sections describe how you can determine for yourself if you have a sleep-breathing condition and what you can do to improve both your sleep quality and overall health.

If you are no longer "on top of your world," if you think that it's your job, or your new family or even your age that is making you sick and tired, you might be surprised to find that it's the way you breath while sleeping that is at the root of all these problems. This concept is the foundation for this book and it may well be your key to a life of renewed energy, vigor, and good health.

Section 1

The New Sleep-Breathing Paradigm

1 Eureka! The Discovery of My Paradigm

I STILL REMEMBER the exact moment it hit me.

I was lying in bed with my wife, Kathy, ready to go to sleep, when I just happened to ask her how she was doing. It had been a very difficult four months since she delivered our second son, Devin.

After our first son, Jonas, who was born three years prior, my wife was extremely tired and depressed for an entire year. All her doctors told her that it was post-partum depression, and that it would eventually go away. It did.

This time it was different. She was not as tired after the second pregnancy, but for four excruciating months, she always felt dizzy and lightheaded, made worse by moving or standing up. Her blood pressure, which was normally on the low side to begin with, was even lower, and at one point the entire right side of her body went numb, which necessitated a visit to the emergency room to ensure she was not having a stroke. She was sent home with a clean bill of health. But clearly, she was not well.

So in answer to that idle question I had asked her that resulted in my "Ah-ha!" experience, she said she was fine. She knew why I was asking her. Pleasantly surprised by her answer, I was curious. "What do you think is the difference that made it go away?"

After a brief moment of reflection, she told me offhandedly, "Well, I did lose all my pregnancy weight."

Then, it hit me. I still vividly remember the light bulb literally flashing on top of my head. It all made sense. I remembered that she had commenced snoring during her third trimester (as many women do), and that her father was diagnosed with obstructive sleep apnea (OSA). I knew that this condition can be hereditary. Obstructive sleep apnea is a sleep-breathing condition where you stop breathing for short periods many times every hour. We know that weight gain can aggravate this condition. Once Kathy had lost her pregnancy weight, she felt much better. In fact, back to how she felt prior to the pregnancy.

But she didn't have obstructive sleep apnea. What she was feeling was something I had just read about in a paper a few weeks earlier. The article discussed young thin women and men who exhibited low blood pressure, experienced lightheadedness and dizziness, and complained of chronic tiredness. These patients did not have OSA but displayed the symptoms of a related but different sleep-breathing condition called upper airway resistance syndrome (UARS). I didn't sleep at all that night.

A few days later, again while in bed after discussing, of all things, how her sleep position had changed as well, another light bulb flicked on. Earlier that day, I had just read an article on the similarity of the timing of heart attacks and the most concentrated time for rapid eye movement (REM) sleep (the dreaming stage). Another scientific paper found that people with OSA are more likely to have heart attacks in the early morning hours (midnight to 6 A.M.), whereas people without OSA are more likely to suffer a heart attack after waking from 6 A.M. to 12 noon.[1]

I was reminded of my days during surgical internship, when an alarming number of otherwise healthy people undergoing routine operations had heart attacks during my early morning shifts. We know that for certain people predisposed to sleep-breathing disorders, sleep position can play a major role in the quality of sleep.

What I realized was that there are some people who prefer to sleep only on their sides or their stomach. Some absolutely cannot sleep on their backs, and must sleep in the latter positions in order to breathe properly. I concluded that what was happening in these situations was that being forced to sleep on their backs for the first time in decades after surgery or another medical procedure resulted in an inability to breathe properly. This, in turn, placed stress on the heart, increasing their risk of heart attack. The critical issue here is that it's during REM sleep that the muscles of the throat are most relaxed. If susceptible people are forced to sleep on their backs, they can no longer adjust in a hospital situation by changing their sleeping position. They are simply forced to sleep on their backs as best they can. This realization led to yet another sleepless night for me. The implications were enormous.

Both these events prompted me to think about other curious things I had observed in the previous few years of practice. Almost every patient with a sleep-breathing problem such as UARS or OSA had some degree of throat acid reflux. Furthermore, many of these same people preferred not to sleep on their backs. The kind of acid reflux that we see in an ear, nose and throat practice is different from the typical heartburn acid reflux, or gastroesophageal reflux disease (GERD). When the acid reaches the throat, it is called laryngopharyngeal reflux disease, or LPRD. In most cases, LPRD is silent, the only symptoms being throat clearing, post-nasal drip, a lump sensation in the throat, hoarseness, cough, choking, or difficulty swallowing. This is probably one of the most common conditions that an ear, nose and throat (ENT) doctor encounters every day.

Interestingly enough, there are numerous studies that show an association between the following pairs of conditions: LPRD and OSA,[2] GERD and asthma,[3] LPRD and chronic sinusitis.[4] In many of these studies, treating the former sometimes, but not always, heals the latter. As I began to research hundreds of articles, I began to see a pattern. In the linked examples given above, LPRD has been shown to be associated with OSA, and LPRD has been shown to be associated with chronic sinusitis, but there appeared to be no cross-linkages, that is, I could find no papers reporting a connection between OSA and chronic sinusitis, for example.

To my amazement, this pattern continued with other non-ENT conditions such as high blood pressure,[5] heart attacks,[5] depression,[6] diabetes,[7] and pre-eclampsia in pregnancy,[8,9] to name a few.

One day, as a simple mental exercise, I wrote down the two most common conditions that I encounter as paired symptoms. These are: acid reflux of the throat and any form of upper airway obstruction. I then spaced the two conditions far apart on a large blank sheet of paper. I drew a curved line with an arrow from one to the other, forming a complete circle (see Figure 1.1). Going back to the research literature, there were numerous papers supporting or suggesting each arrow.

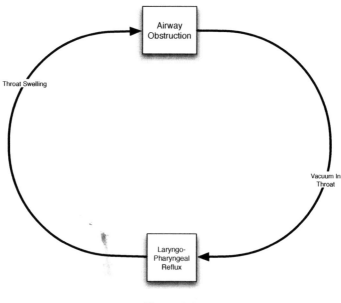

Figure 1.1

For example, with total upper airway obstruction, a tremendous vacuum effect is created in the chest and throat, literally sucking up stomach acid into the throat. There are many other proposed mechanisms for this condition, such as a relaxation of the lower esophageal sphincter, which normally prevents stomach contents from regurgitating into the esophagus. There are also numerous studies that suggest that acid in the throat can aggravate airway collapse merely by numbing the protective airway reflexes present in normal people.[10] These pressure sensors in the throat can detect when there is impending collapse and send a signal to the brain to tighten up throat and tongue muscles.[11]

When acid is present in the throat it can cause more swelling of the delicate surrounding tissues, which promotes additional throat collapse, thus further aggravating this vicious cycle. A recent study suggests that for people who snore, the tremendous soft tissue vibrations caused by snoring can numb or deaden these pressure receptors, worsening any pre-existing upper airway obstruction.

From each of the arrows, I connected arrows to other conditions that came up in my research. Once I "connected" all the dots, the results were truly amazing (see Figure 1.2). What I will describe in the remainder of this chapter is an overly simplified internal physiologic process that can occur within your body as a result of upper airway obstruction and acid reflux in the throat. You may feel a bit overwhelmed by all the lines and arrows in these figures, but rather than focusing on the specific details, concentrate on the "big picture" instead. I will describe only a handful of representative examples in this chapter, and elaborate more in future chapters.

As Figure 1.2 shows, once stomach acid or any other caustic material (such as alkaline bile or pepsin, a digestive enzyme) from the stomach reaches the throat, laryngopharyngeal reflux occurs which promotes swelling of the throat tissues (Arrow 1). In addition, this material can travel down the windpipe and cause swelling and inflammation in the lungs (Arrow 2).

Stomach contents can also move up into the nose, ears, and sinuses (Arrow 3). This can cause swelling and congestion in the nose (Arrow 4), which can further cause a vacuum effect downstream in the throat and increase the potential of throat collapse. Diminished activity in throat pressure receptors due to chronic acid exposure (or vibrations) prevents throat muscle tension during times of collapse, aggravating further collapse (Arrow 5).

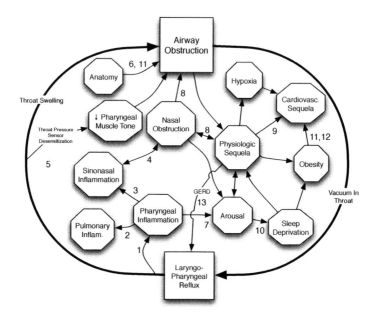

Figure 1.2: A diagrammatic representation of the interconnectedness of various physiologic processes, all precipitated by the vicious cycle of obstruction and throat acid reflux.

Certain anatomic features, such as a small mouth or dental abnormalities, can also accelerate throat collapse (Arrow 6). Acid in the throat can also cause you to wake up frequently in the middle of the night (Arrow 7). These "arousals" can occur consciously or subconsciously. They also prevent you from getting sufficient deep sleep and a restful night.

Arrows 8 shows that nasal and airway obstruction in general results in certain changes in the body's physiology, the end result being lack of oxygen (hypoxia) to the body. Over time, repetitive obstructions and breathing cessations can lead to an internal stress response, leading to cardiovascular complications (Arrow 9). Multiple arousals can lead to sleep deprivation (Arrow 10), which increases stress hormone levels (e.g, cortisol), which makes you eat more and gain weight. Weight gain (Arrow 11) also enlarges the fat cells in your throat and tongue, narrowing the airway, aggravating the original vicious cycle. Weight gain also raises your risk factors for heart disease (Arrow 12).

Finally, certain physiologic factors that involve an imbalance of the involuntary nervous system can lead to loosening of the sphincter that separates the stomach from the esophagus, allowing acid to readily access the throat (Arrow 13).

Hopefully, you'll have your own eureka moment about your fatigue and other health problems as you read through the following chapters.

2 Anatomy 101: Why Humans Choke

I VIVIDLY REMEMBER THE FIRST NIGHT I was on call as a brand new otolaryngology (Ear, Nose and Throat [ENT]) resident, two days fresh from finishing my surgical internship in the mid-90s. I got a STAT (urgent) overhead page to the emergency room (ER). On the phone, the ER nurse relayed frantically that they had a small boy who had a tracheotomy tube that accidentally fell out and they couldn't replace it. He was turning blue and they needed me to come ASAP. A tracheotomy tube is usually used in uncommon situations where there is some type of obstruction in or around the voice box area, such as vocal cord paralysis or papilloma virus growths (in this age-group), or for cancer in older adults. A small hole is surgically made just below the voice-box in the windpipe, and a rigid curved tube is inserted either temporarily or permanently.

I grabbed my fiberoptic camera. This is a long narrow flexible camera, about 4 millimeters (mm) wide. While a stethoscope is a cardiologist's primary diagnostic tool, the ENT specialist instead brandishes his or her fiberoptic device. With one in tow, I ran to the emergency room. It was a large and crowded area and I didn't even know where the boy was. This was a moot point because as soon

11

as I entered, I saw a crowd of about twenty people surrounding a stretcher, with lots of loud orders being called out, and people shuffling in and out from the frantic group. As I approached, one of the nurses recognized me as the ENT resident on call, and screamed out, "Thank God, ENT is here!"

When I saw the huddled mass of doctors, nurses, medical students, respiratory technicians, and others, I took a slow deep breath. I was trembling with fear inside. Besides some basic articles and lectures I had been exposed to about emergency airway situations, I had never managed one before. As I walked closer to the boy, I could hear his struggling high pitched breath sounds. Miraculously, the crowd suddenly began to part, yielding to the expertise of the ENT resident. It was like a scene from the movie, *The Ten Commandments*, when Charlton Heston as Moses parted the Red Sea. Little did they know how little I knew.

After quickly assessing the situation, I realized that the hole had started to close off and tighten, making it difficult to replace the tracheotomy tube. The ER doctors had tried repeatedly and were unable to pass the tube through the neck opening. I took out my fiberoptic camera and quickly looked inside the hole to make sure it was connected properly to the windpipe, which it was. Then instinctively, I passed a small flexible suction tubing into the opening, and threaded the tracheotomy tube over the suction tubing, then slid it down, and with a little force, popped it in place, and then pulled out the suction tubing. This all occurred within a matter of seconds. I could hear sighs of relief around me.

Threading something over a guide-wire is a common technique with many medical procedures. I was fortunate in that I came in later with a fresh objective perspective, and applied a commonly used technique appropriate to this particular situation. Someone else could have easily thought of it as well.

Over the next four years, my fellow ENT residents and I underwent intensive training on how to manage the airway. Some were emergency situations, like the example given above, and others were under more controlled situations, such as upper airway surgery for various ENT conditions, like vocal cord polyps, throat cancer surgery, nasal surgery, pennies in the esophagus, and a range of other conditions.

Later, in private practice, I became very comfortable performing procedures in any part of the upper airway, from the tip of the nose to the windpipe or esophagus. No other medical specialist knows this area inside-out as well as an otolaryngologist does. Facial cosmetic, plastic and reconstructive surgery is also part of our field. Not only are we trained as surgeons in this area, we are also trained as medical doctors for the entire head and neck area, excluding the teeth, brain and eyes. In a sense, we have to be surgeons, allergists, endocrinologists, neurologists, hematologists, rheumatologists, oncologists, pediatricians, and pathologists. In short, we are a regional specialty. It is precisely this broad-based training that provided the key to discover the amazing findings that led me to write this book.

Before I go over some basic anatomy that's relevant to the topic of this book, I want to describe some interesting anatomic concepts and discoveries that serves as the scientific "backbone" of my sleep-breathing paradigm. Finding and reading the following books or papers was another one of the "ah-ha!" moments for me.

There are three anatomic concepts and theories that I find fascinating, and which have profound importance to the concepts described in this book. These findings not only consolidated my paradigm mechanics, but also have frightening implications for all of us.

The first is a comparative anatomy study by Dr. Terrance Davidson in 2003.[1] Based on his own studies of papers published by both comparative anatomists and evolutionary biologists, he presents a convincing argument that with the exception of certain flat-faced dogs, man is the only mammal that has any significant OSA. This is thought to be due to development of complex speech and language skills, which could only occur when the human voice box dropped below the tongue into the neck area.

Davidson notes three anatomic changes that contribute to this phenomenon:

1. Klinorynchy (Figure 2.1): Here the facial skeleton migrates and rotates under the brain cavity. This leads to a narrowing of the breathing passageways and shortening of the facial bones which causes airway narrowing. This is expected, since humans have relatively flattened faces and short facial bones. There's even speculation that because of this skeletal compression, our sinus passageways are more narrow to begin with, predisposing us to sinus infections.

2. Laryngeal descent and loss of the epiglottis–soft palate lock up (Figure 2.2): As a result of "laryngeal descent", the tongue and soft palate tissues became more floppy and pliable. In all other animals (and human infants), the epiglottis (the top-most part of the voice box) touches and overlaps behind the soft palate. But as the voice box descends, a space is created

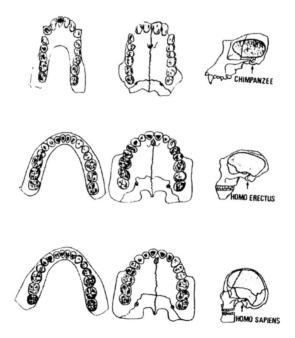

Figure 2.1 Rotation of the facial skeleton down and underneath the skull, and migration of the foramen magnum forward. Note narrowed space between arrow (foramen magnum) and space behind jaws in humans. (From Miles, AEW. The evolution of dentitions in the more recent ancestors of man. [1972]. *Proceedings of the Royal Society of Medicine*, 65(4); 396–399, with permission.)

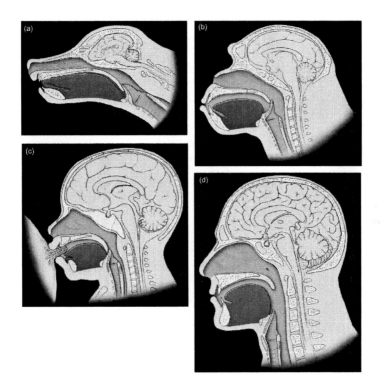

Figure 2.2 Notice how the voice box sits just behind the tongue in animals (a,b) and the human infant (c), but it drops below the tongue in the human adult (arrow, d). Reprinted with permission.[1]

between the soft palate and the epiglottis, which is called the oropharynx (Figure 2.3), and which Davidson states is present only in humans. Human infants are born with a natural suck-swallow-breathing cycle and the elevated epiglottis helps reduce the risk of aspiration of breast milk. As the epiglottis descends to its lower position in later months, the risk of aspiration increases, but by this time, the infant has perfected the act of swallowing.

3. Migration of the foramen magnum (Figure 2.1): This is the opening below the skull that the spinal cord passes through. Notice in the figure that this opening in humans is relatively forward compared to that of a chimpanzee, crowding the already narrowed airway from the shortened facial bones.

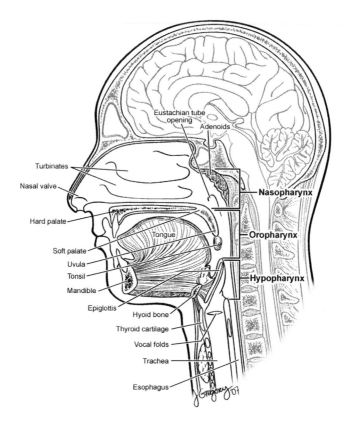

Figure 2.3 Sidewall of nose and throat.

These processes imply that all humans are susceptible to tongue collapse to varying degrees. Since the upper airway has to simultaneously accommodate speech, breathing and swallowing, it's logical that overdevelopment of any one component may be at the expense of the other two. Scientists speculate that speech and language development is ultimately detrimental to the human organism, as evidenced by the fact that only humans can choke on a foreign object and die. Not being able to breathe well when sleeping on our backs may be yet another consequence. It's ironic that this is the price we must pay for complex speech and language development. There are also many variables that can aggravate these events. This is the main focus of this book.

There is another theory in the dental realm which attempts to explain why there are so many sleep-breathing problems in humans in recent years. Dr. Weston Price, a dentist, traveled the world over sixty years ago looking at isolated cultures that lived and ate off the land.[2] He compared their dental health and jaw structures to those who began to eat Western, processed foods. Within one to two generations, these people began to suffer from severe dental caries and misaligned teeth. In addition, people eating Western diets had significant jaw structure narrowing, with major crowding of teeth. In contrast, people living off the land with no Western influences had healthy, vibrant, cavity-free and straight teeth. Their jaws were wide with broad arches, with no crowding whatsoever.

This phenomenon occurred wherever people lived naturally off the land, from the Amazon to the Aborigines in Australia; even on an isolated Gaelic island off the coast of Scotland and the mountain areas of Switzerland, as well with our own Native American populations.

Price also examined many skulls in the burial grounds of ancient cultures and found that there was very little evidence of tooth decay, and the dental arches were wide with no crowding.

It wasn't so much the individual foods they ate, but rather the fact that they ate off the land (or sea), with no processing, preserving or refining whatsoever. Price argued that once these indigenous people started eating Westernized diets, not only did they stop eating foods their teeth were accustomed to chewing, they also suffered a form of malnutrition, contributing to the malformed and cavity-ridden teeth, as well as narrowed arches and dental crowding over time. I suppose that with Western influences, they also contracted and suffered from Western infectious diseases as well.

Third, another dentist, Dr. Brian Palmer, proposed the theory that with the advent of bottle-feeding about 200 years ago, the incidence of sleep-breathing disorders has risen dramatically.[3] Perhaps the abnormal tongue position while suckling on an artificial nipple somehow affects jaw development, or maybe artificially elevated sucking forces prevent proper widening of the infant's delicate jaws.

Regardless of which theory you believe, this is a real problem of epidemic proportions in developed countries around the world. Most dentists will agree that dental crowding and misaligned teeth are rampant these days. It is also interesting to note that only humans get impacted molars.

If all humans have narrowed breathing passageways due to our ability to speak, then it stands to reason that anything that causes further narrowing or blockage along the entire path from the tip of the nose to the voice box can bring on breathing problems at night.

There are two major areas in the throat that can potentially collapse or obstruct: at the palatal level or at the tongue base level (Figure 2.3). You can have obstruction at the tongue level alone, the palate level alone, or both. In many children and adults, the tonsils are so large that they can radically interfere with the breathing process during sleep. This commonly happens during deep or REM sleep. At this point in the sleep cycle, the throat muscles begin to relax and, along with a mild vacuum pressure generated during inspiration, the tonsils cave in inside the throat, causing complete blockage to breathing at the palate level.

In some people, there may be minimal to no tonsils, but the tongue either sits too far back in the throat, or falls back too easily when lying on the back, especially when muscles relax during deep or REM sleep.

Let's say that you are a healthy 25-year-old woman, but over the past few years you've noticed that you don't wake up as refreshed as you used to, and now you need an extra hour of sleep just to get by during the day. You prefer to sleep on your side and sometimes on your stomach. If I were able to look inside your throat, typically, I would see a narrowed space behind your tongue and the back of your throat, which becomes even more narrow when you lay flat on your back (Figure 2.4).

If you happen to start off sleeping on your back, you're fine, as long as you are in light sleep. But as you begin to enter deeper sleep, and your muscles begin to relax, one of three things can happen:

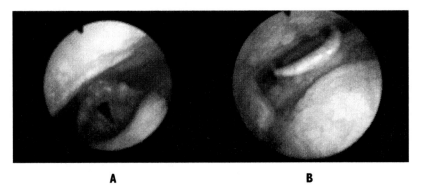

A   **B**

Figure 2.4 Normal wide-open view of voice box in a person sitting up in A, whereas in B, the airway space is very narrowed when lying flat on back.

1. Your tongue falls back only partially. Because you breathe in through your throat at the same rate as through your windpipe, you draw in the air faster against a smaller diameter cross-sectional area, resulting in a vacuum effect upstream in the throat. This causes the area just behind your soft palate to narrow and collapse, making the soft palate flutter and produce snoring noises.
2. Your tongue falls back partially or completely, causing your brain to subconsciously sense that you are about to stop breathing, and wakes you back up to light sleep, starting the cycle over again. Sometimes you wake up completely gasping or choking for air.
3. You obstruct completely, with breathing stoppages lasting from a few seconds to over 30 seconds. Then you wake up.

Which one of the above three scenarios that occurs during sleep determines what kind of health problems you may be susceptible to. Note that you can have any combination of the above three situations.

If you have any other potential source of narrowing, such as with a common cold, allergies, acid reflux, or even weight gain, then even minute amounts of swelling and inflammation will narrow your compromised breathing passageways. This will bring up more stomach contents into the throat, and the entire self-perpetuating vicious cycle begins. If your nose is stuffy even to a slight degree, a mild vacuum effect is created downstream in the throat, and whatever structures that are on the verge of collapsing, do so even more. This in turn causes more obstructions and stomach contents being forced up in your throat, leading to more swelling in the throat and nose, and perpetuation of the vicious cycle.

The combination of speech acquisition, compromised anatomy and upper airway inflammation is a potentially dangerous trio that can not only cause humans to choke occasionally, but can also interrupt breathing while sleeping. This in turn can have serious consequences on your overall health and well-being.

3 Interrupted Breathing, Interrupted Sleep

To put it simply, if you stop breathing, you die. But if you don't breathe well, you get sick. Asthmatics, for example, are unable to pass air through the small diameter air passageways lower down in the lungs. If you've ever had a cold and your nose is stuffy, you will not feel or sleep well. Accidents are also responsible for a range of breathing problems. For example, a small bead that is accidentally aspirated by a young child can lodge in either of the two airway channels called the bronchus, leading to collapse of a lung.

Clearly, the more suddenly that breathing is interrupted, the more urgent the situation. The bead stuck in the child's airway is a great example. In comparison, if you have allergies or mild nasal congestion for two to three weeks, you may be uncomfortable, but you probably would not go to the emergency room.

Most of us take breathing for granted: It's something that is done automatically, even when you are not consciously thinking about it. When you are aware and thinking about your breathing and make an effort to slow down or increase your rate of breathing, then you have overridden the involuntary nervous system and activated your voluntary nervous system. This can be used to your advantage, as we'll discover in a later chapter.

All of this is obvious. Problems arise, however, while you are sleeping. There are six stages of sleep: awake, stage 1, stage 2, stage 3, stage 4, and REM (rapid eye movement) (see Figure 3.1). REM sleep is better known as the "dreaming" stage, stages 1 and 2 are the "light" stages of sleep, and stages 3 and 4 are the "deep" or delta stages of sleep. We need a good distribution of all the sleep stages for proper restorative sleep. Notice how one can cycle up and down the different stages for a total of three to four cycles during sleep. REM sleep is more common near the end of the night. This is why you sometimes remember your dreams vividly, especially when you happen to wake up during the REM phase of sleep.

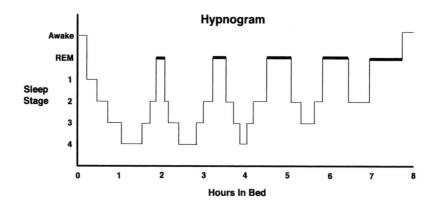

Figure 3.1: Typical hypnogram. Notice 4–5 cycles throughout the night with longer periods of deep (stage 3 and 4) sleep earlier and more REM later during the entire sleep period.

Until recently, many people had an unfortunate stereotypical belief about sleep—that it is a time for "turning off" the body and brain to recharge and prepare for the upcoming day. We now know that sleep is an active and necessary process that is critical to the quality of the following day as well. Whenever you have too much or too little of any of the sleep stages, then you will feel it in the morning, and for the rest of the day. I will discuss how to optimize your sleep quality later in this book.

During the deep stages of sleep, and especially during REM sleep, all the muscles in your body relax, except for your diaphragm, so you can keep breathing. A switch in your brain automatically turns on the signal that relaxes all the muscle activity in your body, including the throat and tongue muscles. One common theory is that if this didn't happen, you could physically act out your dreams and hurt yourself or someone else. There are certain sleep disorders where a faulty switch allows this to happen.

Due to the anatomic factors that I discussed in the prior chapter, for some people who are more susceptible, problems can arise when you are in deep sleep (or REM sleep), and when you are on your back. Since all humans are susceptible to the tongue collapsing to various degrees, given the same situation, different people will obstruct more than others.

For example, if you have no problem sleeping on your back and you get a simple cold, your nose gets stuffed up and due to the vacuum pressures that are created downstream, your tongue can start to fall back, causing you to wake up frequently. This is the reason why you toss and turn when you have a cold. But once your cold goes away, you can catch up on your sleep, and you feel fine again.

Pregnant women, especially in the third trimester, typically don't sleep well. This is not only because of the lack of mobility associated with the pregnancy itself, but also due to increased fat deposits in the throat at this time. The latter serves to narrow the airway, and creates breathing problems that did not exist prior to pregnancy.

If you are young and healthy, and are comfortable sleeping on your back, then continue to do so. However, as you age, the throat tissues start to sag, especially if you gain weight. When this occurs, your throat and tongue tissues may collapse, disrupting your deep sleep.

For those people who are susceptible to tongue collapse during deep sleep while lying on their backs, many automatically adjust and compensate by sleeping on their sides or stomachs. Some people don't know why—they just have a preference. Others absolutely cannot sleep on their backs. This is typically done subconsciously, so you may not realize this is happening. Problems begin when narrowing and obstruction start to occur even while sleeping on the side or stomach.

Let's imagine that you are about to fall asleep on your back. As you go into light sleep you are breathing well, until you enter deep sleep, and due to muscle relaxation, your tongue begins to fall back slightly. This small amount of airflow resistance to breathing is sensed by your brain and it tells your body to wake up, tensing your muscles, to prevent a total breathing occlusion. So the brain "wakes up" somewhat to light sleep. Alternatively, you may wake up completely. Sometimes the tongue falls back and obstructs completely and you wake up gasping or choking, occasionally in a state of panic. Over time, after weeks of tossing and turning, you consciously or subconsciously realize that you can fall asleep much faster if you sleep on your side.

During this entire process, you may or may not snore. If your soft palate is normal with no relaxation or redundancy, then you probably won't. If you have an excess of soft palate tissue and it's a little lax, then as the tongue falls back lightly, due to increased upstream airflow, a greater vacuum effect is created. Think about sucking in through a thin flimsy straw. As you suck in harder, the straw will collapse. If you slowly pinch the middle of the straw, the other end will collapse. If you pinch the end, then the middle will collapse. Most of us learned this as kids, but the same phenomenon can be applied to our breathing apparatus. This basic principle of physics causes the tissues around the back of the soft palate to narrow, and the soft palate may begin to flutter, leading to snoring (see Chapter 21).

Whether your tongue falls back partially or completely, what happens next depends on the state of your throat's nervous system feedback loop. There are pressure sensors in the throat that can detect if there is an impending obstruction. If these receptors are working and intact, then signals go to your brain telling you to wake up and tense your throat muscles to keep it open. If these pressure sensors don't work properly, then your tongue will fall back and eventually obstruct your breathing completely.

In the above situation, one of two things may happen: You can have a conscious or subconscious arousal (to awake or light sleep), or you can stop breathing completely for up to thirty to forty seconds. Depending on how quickly you are taken out of deep sleep, versus how long you stop breathing determines your quality of sleep and, ultimately, the nature of the symptoms you experience by day.

If breathing stops completely (apnea) or there exists significant diminished breathing due to partial obstruction (hypopnea) for more than ten seconds at a time, and if there are more than fifteen of these events every hour (the AHI or apnea hypopnea index), this is officially what is called OSA. It's estimated that about 4% of men and 2% of women in this country have this condition using the above criteria.[1] Using looser, more realistic criteria (over five events every hour with signs or symptoms such as daytime fatigue, high blood pressure, heart disease, or depression), this figure goes up significantly to 24% in men and 9% in women. Obviously this can only be determined by undergoing a formal overnight sleep study.

OSA was first described in the 1960s in older heavy-set men who snored and had a history of falling asleep during the day. Back in medical school and even today, whenever the topic of OSA is brought up in a lecture, the speaker almost always shows a picture of Joe the Fat Boy from Dickens's *The Posthumous Papers of the Pickwick Club* (Figure 3.2). What we now know is that this stereotypical image is just the extreme end of the spectrum, and doctors now believe it may even be a different condition altogether.

Unfortunately, most doctors still have that picture in their minds, and never even think about OSA, especially if the patient is female, thin, or doesn't complain of severe snoring. In fact, it's been shown recently that young thin women who don't snore can have significant OSA. I have many patients like this in my practice.

Untreated OSA has been proven to lead to high blood pressure, and there are numerous studies showing significant increased risks for diabetes, obesity, depression, heart disease, erectile dysfunction, heart attack and stroke. I am amazed how often I see patients who actually fit the stereotypical apnea patient, complete with high blood pressure, diabetes, depression, history of heart attack, and severe snoring, and the thought of OSA is never even considered by the

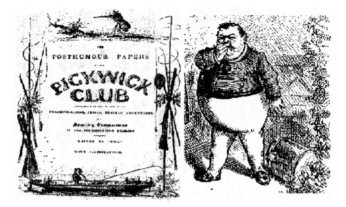

Figure 3.2: Joe the Fat Boy from Dickens's novel, *The Posthumous Papers of the Pickwick Club.*

primary care physician. It is estimated that this condition remains undiagnosed in 80% of men and 90% of women in this country.[2]

One of the challenges in the field of sleep medicine is that no one really knows what the cutoff level is for OSA. In children, the current number is one episode per hour. If your young daughter stops breathing more than once every hour for ten seconds or more, there are many good papers that suggest she should be treated. In adults, the official minimal cutoff line is 5. So if your 17-years and 364 day-old son has an AHI of 4, when he turns 18 the following day, he is officially an adult and no longer has OSA. This is the problem with test results involving thresholds. There's not much difference between 4.9 and 5.1, so officially, one person can have OSA and the other not.

Ideally, the AHI number should be as low as possible. But there are many normal people with mild levels of OSA who function just fine, whereas others have relatively similar numbers but are severely affected by the condition. At the other extreme, there are people with severe OSA (with AHI levels in the 50s to 60s) who don't experience any adverse symptoms. Similar to high blood pressure or high cholesterol where symptoms are largely absent, elevated levels of apneas also raises the risk of heart disease. The bottom line is that it is not the number, but rather the patient, that is important. Examining the entire medical, social and family history is essential and there is no absolute treatment recommendation based on numbers alone.

One of the ways we overcome the above shortcoming is to determine what kind of problems the patient is experiencing, and what medical conditions are present. The patient may have mild OSA, but if the patient does not complain of symptoms and no medical conditions are present, it may be difficult to justify any form of treatment. Knowing that an AHI of 6–7 has been demonstrated to significantly increase the risk of high blood pressure compared with numbers below 5, what do you recommend to such a person? This debate is currently raging in the sleep medicine scientific and research community and presents ethical as well as practical challenges.

Another frustrating situation occurs in patients who don't officially qualify as having apneas or hypopneas. For example, if you stop breathing thirty times every hour, but each episode lasts for only nine seconds, you will be told you don't have OSA. There are probably large numbers of people who fit this criterion, many more than would experience OSA. This former group doesn't have heart disease, but displays various other conditions, such as being tired all the time, being prone to recurrent infections, strange aches and pains, headaches, etc.

This is where the newly described condition called UARS comes in. It was first described by one of the pioneers in sleep medicine, Dr. Christian Guilleminault at Stanford University in the early 1990s.[3] He originally studied chronically tired young men and women who underwent overnight sleep studies and were found to fall outside of the official criteria for OSA. Traditionally, unless another good reason for their fatigue was found, they were given the diagnosis of "idiopathic hypersomnia," meaning we doctors have no idea why they are tired.

Upon more careful analysis, Dr. Guilleminault found that this group all experienced multiple "arousals" during deep sleep, preventing them from maintaining consistent deep sleep. He used pressure sensitive catheters in these patients' throats to measure the negative chest pressures while attempting to breathe in with the throat closed off. What he described was obstruction followed by two or three gradually stronger inspiratory efforts, ending in an arousal, which prevented them from staying in deep sleep. These episodes were only a few seconds long, not meeting the official criteria for an apnea. Nevertheless, he treated them just as if they had OSA and almost all patients reported improvement.

Additional studies show that these patients exhibit other common features such as cold hands, dizziness and lightheadedness, low blood pressure, and orthostatic intolerance.[4] The latter term refers to the dizziness, lightheadedness and occasional short blackouts experienced upon standing up too quickly. Here, the confused nervous system can't react quickly enough to tighten the blood vessels leading to the brain, hence the familiar symptoms. About a quarter of UARS patients were found to have low blood pressure.

Another study observed that UARS patients tended to have more sleep onset insomnia, headaches, temporomandibular joint disease (TMJ), depression, gastroesophageal reflux disease (GERD), runny nose, hypothyroidism, and asthma compared with OSA patients.[5] They found that more women had UARS, together with a higher incidence of sleep onset insomnia, migraine headaches, irritable bowel syndrome, and "alpha-delta" sleep as compared to males. Alpha-delta sleep is typically associated with the "somatic" syndromes, such as chronic fatigue syndrome (CFS), fibromyalgia, depression, and irritable bowel syndrome (IBS). Alpha waves are faster brain waves which are typically present when you are awake and relaxed, with your eyes closed. Delta sleep includes slower wave sleep stages 3 and 4. So when "awake" alpha brain waves intrude into deep-sleep delta waves, this is termed alpha-delta sleep. People displaying alpha-delta sleep waves commonly report unrefreshing sleep and chronic fatigue.

Even before I came across these papers, I was observing similar findings. Coupled with a recent landmark study that showed that most "sinus" headaches are actually migraine attacks in the sinuses, it all made sense.

Here's an example: Sally is a 27-year-old accountant who came to see me after suffering from multiple sinus infections over the past few months. She had completed several courses of antibiotics, and had tried various allergy medications and decongestants, with only temporary relief. She stated that her condition began as a "cold" with a scratchy and painful throat. This later turned into a cough, and subsequently traveled to her ears and sinuses, resulting in sinus headaches which were unbearable. Her nose alternated between being constantly runny or stuffy. She claimed to have been chronically tired all the time, but in the past few months she had found it difficult even getting out of bed. She reported that she felt like she'd only slept for two hours, rather than the entire night. Sally is 5' 3" and of thin build.

I then questioned Sally about her other symptoms, prior to when her sinus problems developed. Even back then, she admitted that she was "tired of being tired," and never felt completely rested when she woke in the morning. Currently, she has trouble falling asleep, and frequently wakes in the middle of the night because she's a light sleeper. Her husband's snoring compounded the problem. Sally also noted that she had just changed jobs and found the process very stressful. Every little thing now bothers her at work and at home, and she finds herself snapping at people over trivial matters.

She also reported that for as long as she can remember, she only feels comfortable sleeping on her stomach, and rarely on her sides. She has chronically cold hands and feet, and has to sleep with socks, even in the summer. She's recently gained about five pounds that she finds hard to lose as she's too tired to exercise. Her diet is not particularly healthy either. Her blood pressure is usually low, and consequently she often feels faint and dizzy when she stands up too quickly.

Sally also has a history of asthma, together with extended episodes of chronic diarrhea that can last for weeks to months, typically brought on by eating certain foods, or as a result of stress. She gets frequent colds and infections, which linger for weeks at a time.

Her father also has a history of heavy snoring, is currently clinically depressed, has high blood pressure, and suffered a heart attack at age 49. Her mother is overweight, snores sometimes, and has diabetes. Her younger brother has ADHD (attention deficit hyperactivity disorder) for which he takes Ritalin, a drug commonly used for ADHD sufferers. Sally feels that her life is falling apart, and she perceives herself as "an old maid." Her doctor recommended that she take a medication for her anxiety condition.

When I examined Sally, I found that her nasal turbinates were swollen (see Chapter 2 on anatomy). She had no tonsils, as they were removed at the age of five. I found it difficult to examine the back of her throat because her tongue was large, impeding the use of a tongue depressor. When I was able get a glimpse of her throat, it was quite narrow.

When I asked her to lie flat on her back (using a tiny flexible camera), her tongue fell almost completely to the back of her mouth, leaving a small slit between the tongue and the back of her throat through which to breathe. I wasn't able to see the voice box at all. When she pushed her lower jaw forward, her tongue moved forward, and I could see one-half of her voice-box, which showed that the back part was irritated and swollen (see Figure 3.3). This confirmed her previous history of repeated chronic throat clearing and post-nasal drip.

Now compare the above example with the following: A 55-year-old woman who came to see me because she was embarrassed by her snoring when she goes on trips. She currently weighs 165 pounds, compared with the 120 pounds she weighed back in her early twenties. She takes medication for both high blood pressure and depression. She noted that in her twenties she used to have cold hands and feet, but is no longer troubled by this. Her blood pressure used to be low back then as well, but now it's high, hence the blood pressure medication. She is at the tail end of menopause, and she reported that much of the transition was difficult. She has gained additional weight since menopause and also finds herself nodding off at important office meetings.

What I described in the first example is a young thin woman with UARS, whereas the second woman probably has OSA. The second

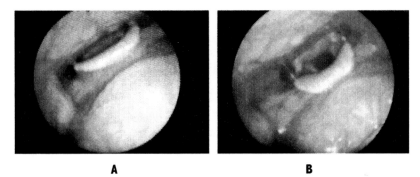

Figure 3.3: Note narrow airway opening while lying flat (A), and significant increase in airway diameter after jaw thrust maneuver (B).

woman could easily be the first woman, only 28 years older. More often than not, I see this pattern happening repeatedly.

One exception to the rule is when a person who doesn't have any problems sleeping on their back begins to gain significant weight—over 25–50 pounds. Under these circumstances, the person tends to have more palatal narrowing and a lesser degree of tongue collapse, so there is no significant sleep position preference.

What I have observed over many years can be best understood by using a sleep-breathing continuum concept (Figure 3.4). Think of it as a diagonal line with normal people near the left side of the line, UARS people near the middle and OSA people on the right side. If you catch a cold, the accompanying breathing obstruction while sleeping, comprising multiple arousals or apneas, makes you feel tired and miserable during the day. When the cold goes away, everything returns to normal. On the curve, you have temporarily slid up the line to the right, but revert to your original position once the cold is gone. But if you slide up and never come back down, you'll feel chronically tired and never wake up refreshed.

Pregnant women, by this definition, are often miserable in their third trimesters because they slide up the line due to weight gain. Some women never lose all the pregnancy weight, and this can lead to problems (see Chapter 12). If you are at the extreme right of the

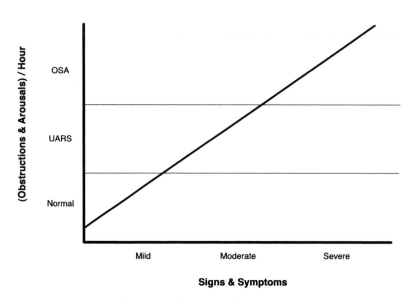

Figure 3.4: Sleep-breathing continuum

line, then you'll have OSA, where you stop breathing many times for greater than ten seconds per episode.

What I've noticed is that if you slide up the scale and remain there, after several months or years you will adjust to your new upper airway, and you won't feel as bad as you used to in the past. Even when you go back down the slope to the left, you can feel the difference. The key concept here is that only when you are actively moving up or down the line, do you feel more tired or fatigued. Once you stop moving, you'll feel better, but only back to your elevated baseline condition.

Other factors that facilitate movement up or down the line include stress, colds, allergies or infections, and weight change. These will be discussed in subsequent chapters.

4   **Why Sleep Position Matters**

BACK IN MEDICAL SCHOOL, I remember seeing part of a video from a study that revealed that all normal people move about frequently in bed. Anyone who regularly has the chore of making their own or their children's beds knows this intuitively. But why do we have certain positional preferences, and why do we need to move around? Evolutionary biologists claim that primitive humans evolved their sleep cycles (light, deep and REM sleep) to prevent staying permanently in deep sleep, and intermittently cycling through stages of lighter sleep, in order to be vigilant against predators. If you have ever watched a dog "asleep" you will immediately understand this process. Dogs may seem to be asleep but they are easily woken. Yet at other times, we can observe them undergoing REM sleep, complete with flickering eyelids and even body movements and muffled barks.

The one sure thing is that most of us move around and roll over in bed to various degrees throughout the course of the night. Some of us have a preference for one specific position, and others absolutely must sleep in another.

From a sleep-breathing standpoint, sleep position is critical. As discussed in the anatomy chapter, your upper airway anatomy predisposes you to certain sleep positions that are more optimal than others.

There are four basic positions: back, right side, left side, and stomach. Stop reading for a few seconds and think about what your favorite position is, or in which position you think you sleep most of your nights. I'm willing to bet that many of you have a preference. If you don't know, or if you sleep in all four positions, then ask your bed-partner. Some people never find any position comfortable to sleep in for any extended length of time, and as a result toss and turn all night long, never getting a sufficient amount of deep, restful sleep.

If you recall what was described in the prior chapter on anatomy, the need for some people to sleep in certain positions is clear: Due to various degrees of facial skeletal flattening or narrowing, along with the concept of laryngeal descent, the human tongue is susceptible to collapse backwards under certain conditions. This occurs most commonly when you sleep on your back, mainly due to gravity. It's been shown that astronauts with OSA have fewer difficulties with this condition while in space, without the influence of gravity.[1]

Even if your facial and throat anatomy is completely normal, whenever you catch a bad cold and your nose gets stuffy, one of the reasons you'll toss and turn at night and can't sleep well is because your tongue keeps falling back. Every time you go into deep sleep, the muscles in your throat begin to relax, and during inspiration, your tongue falls back and obstructs breathing. This particularly occurs whenever you are on your back. You'll keep waking up, repeatedly being taken out of deep to light sleep. Once your cold goes away, and sleep loss is restored, you are fine once again. Similarly, the weight gain that accompanies the latter stages of pregnancy results in additional complications if you should catch a cold. The increased fat reserves in the throat, together with cold symptoms such as a blocked or runny nose, make for a poor sleeping experience.

For anyone with a narrow or small oral cavity, the tongue is much more susceptible to falling back. Many people in this situation find it much easier to fall asleep on their sides, or sometimes on their stomachs. But because of the baseline amount of narrowing, a simple cold or allergy attack can disrupt sleep significantly via the following mechanism. Take for example, John, after a bad allergy attack with a stuffy nose, who normally sleeps on his side, finds it difficult to fall asleep, and feels tired and foggy-headed even after sleeping for a good eight hours. As described in the previous chapter, stomach contents can be sucked up into the throat silently, causing additional irritation and swelling resulting in further collapse, and so the process continues. This is a vicious cycle that has the capability to extend a simple cold into a semi-chronic condition that can last for weeks to months. Furthermore, acid or bile from the stomach can also leak into the windpipe and lungs, causing further irritation and inflammation in both these locations. Once acid reaches the throat it can go in any direction including the lungs, nose, sinuses and ears.

Due to intermittent stomach content exposure and incorrect messages received by the involuntary nervous system governing the nasal region, the membranes remain chronically swollen. Nasal mucous membranes swell up and extra mucous is created due to an overreaction on the part of the immune and nervous systems, and nasal problems result. Even minor nasal congestion can aggravate tongue collapse. This can cause a true post-nasal drip, which really originates from the nose, rather than from the mucous secreting glands of the throat. The initial throat irritation (from acid) can seem like the beginning of a cold, but no fever develops, and later the problem may travel up into the ears, and lastly into the nose and sinuses (Figure 2.3). If you look at the side-wall of the nose again you'll see why the ears are more commonly affected in this situation than the sinuses. Due to gravity, it's easier for stomach contents to reach the Eustachian tube, whereas to reach the sinus passageways, the stomach contents must take a right angled turn and move up towards the front of the nose, where the sinus openings are located.

Unfortunately, in this situation many people are prescribed oral antibiotics when there is no evidence of a bacterial infection.

Fortunately, most people compensate very well without needless drugs, only experiencing intermittent "colds" and "infections," until something happens that forces them to sleep for extended periods on their back.

After starting to sleep on her back, one young woman told me that that was when her body started to "fall apart." I often hear stories such as this from my patients. Another situation which highlights problems associated with sleeping position is when you are sick or have to be hospitalized, which in most cases, forces you to sleep on your back, due to the presence of wires, monitor leads, etc. Most people find it difficult to be forced to sleep solely on their back, and sleep better once they are able to assume their position of choice after returning home.

People who have a chronic injury, such as a hip or shoulder problem, also can't roll around freely in bed and are not able to sleep well for months or even years. To complicate matters, immobility during sleep coupled with hormonal influences from inefficient sleep can result in weight gain. The added weight narrows the throat, narrowing the airway even further. Even if you can sleep quite comfortably on your side or stomach, something as simple as a toe injury that prevents you from staying active or exercising normally can promote weight gain as well.

In fact, if you have pain in any area of your body, it can be of sufficient intensity to wake you up during the night. But consider this: Maybe it's poor sleep efficiency that is causing you to be more sensitive to the pain, which then promotes frequent wakening.[2]

In addition, if you are continually prevented from staying in deep sleep, then any little pinch or discomfort while in bed can easily wake you. This may be where improved mattress technology can play a role.

The situation is even more pronounced in a hospital setting. I described my experiences in my surgical internship in a previous chapter, particularly my bewilderment as to why so many relatively healthy people suffered unexpected heart attacks on my shift at five in the morning.

Let's say that you are a man in your sixties going into a hospital for a routine hip operation. You're a little overweight, and you take medications for your high blood pressure and high cholesterol. The operation goes smoothly, and the pain is manageable. That first night after the surgery, you can't sleep at all in the beginning. Finally, once you are able to fall asleep, you wake up around 6 A.M. having trouble breathing and your chest is tight, with pain shooting down your left arm.

You've just had a heart attack. Luckily, it was a mild one and you'll recover. But over the next few days, the breathing problem doesn't get much better and you start to cough. When you start having fevers, the surgeon orders a chest x-ray, which reveals pneumonia. After treatment for this infection, you finally go home. After a few weeks of rehabilitation, you're back to work again. But compared to how you felt before the operation, you're below par, and feel tired all the time, despite sleeping for eight hours each night. You blame it on having gained about ten pounds since the operation.

I see similar situations all the time in my practice. Someone who is a side or stomach sleeper does so to compensate for tongue collapse. Suddenly, they are forced to sleep on their back after undergoing surgery. A hospital bed is not conducive to sleeping on either the sides of the body or the stomach. Besides being interrupted every hour or so for vitals and other nursing duties, the head of the bed is usually tilted up somewhat, and you'll have one or more intravenous lines or other devices connected to your body, effectively preventing you from sleeping the way you prefer.

Not only is it hard for you to fall asleep on your back, but once you do, you keep waking up whenever you start to enter deep sleep, due to relaxation of your throat muscles. When you enter REM sleep, your throat muscles are at their most relaxed state, and at this point you are most prone to complete breathing obstruction. If obstruction occurs and persists for more than ten to thirty seconds for anywhere between twenty to one hundred times an hour, there may be serious repercussions. Under these circumstances, the heart is deprived of oxygen, and this can lead to chest pain, breathing difficulties and, ultimately, a heart attack.

We know that most heart attacks occur during the early morning hours. Coincidentally, this is also the time that we experience our longest REM (dream) periods. If you already have a weakened heart, even minor pauses in breathing can facilitate a heart attack .

Just to complicate matters, if you just had surgery and are in pain, you're usually given a narcotic pain medication. Narcotics are known to diminish breathing, and potentially numb the protective airway reflexes that alert the brain to the presence of an obstruction.

Furthermore, once the throat is partially or completely blocked, the vacuum pressures that build up in the throat can literally suck up acid or other stomach contents into the throat. This material can travel into the lungs or up into the nose. The patient referred to above probably suffered from what is known as aspiration pneumonia. Acid is very caustic to the lungs. No wonder people have so many complications in a hospital.

Until now, the significance of sleep position has been described only in the psychology literature and the lay press as models for predicting personality types. However, not only can the sleep-breathing paradigm predict certain personality types based on sleep position (as it relates to sleep deprivation and stress states), but it can also provide clues about our mental and physical state of health and disease.

Section 2

The Many Facets of the Sleep-Breathing Paradigm

This section describes various medical conditions that we take for granted as independent conditions (see Figure below). Don't be intimidated by the lines and figures. You've seen the main circle before in Chapter 2. The main point of this figure is to illustrate the complexity of the body's processes and how they are intimately connected. Viewed from the sleep-breathing paradigm, many, if not most of these conditions are all linked or interrelated. Each of the arrows entering or exiting the central "intrinsic area" (physiologic processes) are either documented in the scientific literature, or represent a link that makes common sense (e.g. changing your nasal anatomy can cause nasal obstruction). The "extrinsic" shapes are conditions (squares) or symptoms (ovals) that are either a result of the intrinsic processes or contribute into the central "intrinsic" factors. Selected symptoms and medical conditions are discussed in the coming chapters.

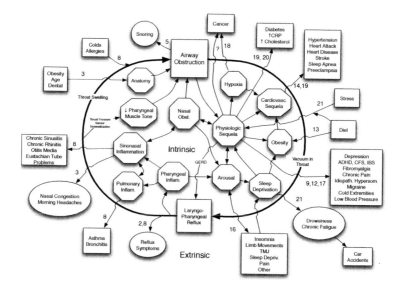

The Sleep-Breathing Paradigm. Numbers next to arrows represent corresponding chapters that describe the link. Not all conditions are described in the chapters.

5 Creativity, Stress & Breathing

Jason is a sculptor who works as an administrative assistant during the day and came to see me due to recurrent sinus infections. He normally sculpts at night. He snores, sleeps only on his stomach, and keeps odd hours, usually going to bed around 1–2 A.M. He never feels refreshed in the morning, no matter how long he sleeps. He states that whenever he goes through periods of not being able to produce, he deliberately sleep-deprives himself in order to enhance his creativity.

IF YOU DON'T GET ENOUGH SLEEP, you will be tired and cranky, and being tired can affect your mood. As described in prior chapters, poor breathing at night while sleeping can definitely affect the quality of your sleep. But what does being tired have to do with your level of creativity? Let's look at our sleep-breathing continuum (see Figure 5.1). Normal people are at the lower left hand side of the line, with no obvious sleep-breathing issues, and at the far right are people with OSA. People with upper airway resistance syndrome are somewhere in the middle. Moving upwards and to the right

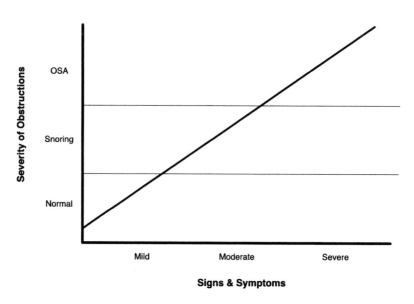

Figure 5.1 Sleep-breathing continuum

indicates that your body is under low-grade, but continuous state of stress.

Over the years, I've noticed a definite pattern in a person's occupation and the presence of sleep-breathing disorders. In particular, I've noticed in my practice that people in creative fields such as writers, artists or musicians tend to have mild UARS. I don't think I'm over-generalizing when I say that some creative types tend to keep odd hours to accommodate their unpredictable schedules. They also engage in episodic bursts of creative activity and energy, usually prompted by the stresses of deadlines and major performances.

People with UARS tend to be tired more often than not. It doesn't matter how long they sleep—they never wake up fully refreshed, even after 8–9 hours of sleep. Usually they will attribute their fatigue to their unpredictable schedules and stressful lives. Not sleeping long enough adds to the problem. This begs the question, does having a creative career lead to fatigue, or does the fatigue itself (aided by UARS) lead to, or enhance creativity?

It's been shown in many sleep deprivation studies that people who don't sleep well are in a physiologic state of stress. An extreme example of stress would be if you were being chased by a tiger. This is a life-or-death emergency, and your primary concern would be to run away as quickly as possible from the tiger. In a split second, your involuntary nervous system has to react instantly to assist you to run away.

Your involuntary nervous system is made up of two components: the sympathetic and the parasympathetic nervous systems. The sympathetic, or "fight or flight" response, speeds up your heart rate, increases your blood pressure, and activates your entire nervous system to prepare to fight or run away. In this situation, adrenaline is released, as well as many other signaling chemical messengers that tell your body to prepare to do battle. It also diverts blood, energy and resources away from less necessary body areas such as your gastrointestinal system, your reproductive organs, your skin and your extremities, to more important areas such as your central muscles, your heart and your brain.

The parasympathetic nervous system controls the opposite response. This part of your involuntary nervous system involves the long-term investment activities that the body needs to digest food, store energy, reproduce, or sleep.

Normally, your involuntary nervous system is on autopilot, each component being gradually turned on or off like a delicate physiologic seesaw. However, if for whatever reason your stress response is activated such that it assumes a long-term, low-grade level, then a certain series of events can occur. This happens whether you are being chased by a tiger or thinking about your taxes. If you keep waking up due to mild tongue collapse, this causes you not to sleep well, since you can't maintain long periods of deep sleep. This can lead to a chronic, low-grade stress response within your body.

There are also many studies that suggest that sleep deprivation can lower a person's pain threshold. This means that a sleep deprived person will sense pain a lot earlier and a lot more magnified for the same amount of pain compared with a person who sleeps well. If pain is a form of sensory input from your skin to your brain, then in theory, all the other forms of sensory input, including general sensation, taste, hearing, smell, vision, and maybe even our emotions, can potentially be heightened with any degree of sleep deprivation.

Remember the last time you were in a haunted house, or watching a scary movie, or even if you were ever on a deserted street at night in the middle of a dangerous neighborhood? In all these situations, all your senses are heightened in order for you to anticipate any real or perceived forms of danger. Under such circumstances, you can hear everything, even a pin drop. I'm sure you will have also heard of people who claim that a certain odor or sound brings up disturbing memories of a traumatic event suffered in the past.

Here's another chicken or the egg question: Is a stock trader (or any other intense and stressful profession working long and crazy hours) tired all the time because of stress and lack of sleep, or is lack of sleep and stress making him work long and crazy hours so he can stay awake? One of the most common situations that I see is when people with sleep-breathing problems quit their boring desk jobs and find a more high intensity, stimulating profession, where they move around all the time, interacting with people constantly. These same people tend to seek out jobs, activities or hobbies that keep them focused and awake. They are miserable working at jobs that require longs periods of inactivity. If they still have one of these jobs, they are intense athletes after work, sometimes to the point of being addicted. Many people tell me that they have to exercise intensely for 1–2 hours every day. If they skip even one or two days, they feel tired and lethargic.

These are the same people who also can't sleep on their backs. Frequently, if they injure themselves to the point where they can't maintain the intensity of their workouts for weeks or months, they begin to gain weight, which narrows their throats, causing further tongue collapse, nudging them progressively up the sleep-breathing continuum.

Once they start to slide up the sleep-breathing continuum line, they also start moving further away from the midline on the sleep-breathing continuum. Any advantage or talent they had with their heightened senses now begins to turn detrimental, where a simple odor that used to be pleasing is now a noxious fume, or a certain tone or sound can be irritating, almost to the point of disability.

Stress can come from the inside (physiologic or the sleep-breathing arousal mechanism), as well as from any "outside" source, including psychological, emotional or physical. Your body does not care where the stress is coming from. It will react the same way regardless of its origin. Another point is that people are much more symptomatic while they are moving up the continuum line. Once they stop moving, their bodies adjust, and they start to feel "normal" again (back to their baseline condition). So anything that pushes them up the line (internal or external stress, mild weight gain, colds, allergies, infections, sleep position changes) can accelerate the vicious self-perpetuating cycle. In other words, any relative change in a person's sleep-breathing status can produce symptoms.

Many people can also pinpoint the exact time that they began to feel overwhelmingly tired with an inability to achieve deep sleep and wake up refreshed in the morning. There is usually a precipitating event, such as a bad infection, injury, pregnancy or an intensely stressful event (death, divorce, etc.). Imagine if this state continued for months or years, think how it would adversely affect you in your daily activities, your job, and in your personal life.

What this suggests is that creativity may be a uniquely human characteristic that is a natural consequence of complex speech and language development. Yet this heightened sense of awareness and creativity, taken to the extreme, can also be detrimental. Various degrees of deep sleep deprivation could also not only affect your mood or temperament, but determine your chosen hobby or occupation. In this context, mild sleep deprivation may be necessary for certain forms of human creativity.

6

Common Ear, Nose & Throat Problems: What You May Not Know

Jane is 24 and seems to suffer from sinus infections almost on a monthly basis. She has taken 6–7 courses of oral antibiotics in the past year. Every time she catches a cold, it turns into a major infection with pain, headaches, nasal congestion and post-nasal drip. Even weather changes can aggravate her infections.

EAR, SINUS AND THROAT INFECTIONS make up a major portion of routine visits to doctors. All too often an antibiotic is prescribed, not based on clinical skill or reason, but more for convenience. It's easier and quicker to prescribe an antibiotic than to take the time to educate the patient on why prescribing an antibiotic is not the way to treat most of these conditions. It seems like much of what we learned in medical school is thrown out the window when we doctors enter the real world of practicing medicine.

We're all taught that antibiotics are useful only for treating bacterial infections. Even the lay press and media outlets warn repeatedly that antibiotics are useless for simple colds, which are caused by viruses. Despite all this information, antibiotics usage has not decreased; if anything, it's increased. Resistance to many antibiotics is rising mostly due to overprescribing by physicians. Part of this is fueled by direct to consumer advertising that was recently approved by the government. Our airwaves are inundated with commercials touting the advantages and benefits of taking a pill for every symptom that exists. This can make for some demanding patients, asking for a certain medication based on a commercial.

Furthermore, it's not just viral infections that are being inappropriately treated with antibiotics—symptoms of allergies and acid reflux are also frequently treated with antibiotics, usually with no effect. But because some patients feel better in a few days, they attribute their improvement to the pills. In most cases, they would have felt better just with conservative treatment. However, in many other cases, the symptoms don't improve and patients are given another stronger round of antibiotics. Sometimes they are given the same antibiotic. Not uncommonly, patients are given the wrong type of antibiotic that is essentially useless for the presumed type of bacterial infection that is being treated. The problem remains.

At this point, patients are then referred to an ENT specialist, like me. Usually the patient has been suffering from chronic throat pain for the past few weeks. Interestingly, a patient history often reveals that there was no fever, chills, colored discharge, sneezing, chills, or cough. Only a sore throat, and typically on one side of the throat.

Our bodies come complete with harmless bacteria living in the nose and throat cavity. Only when specific strains of bacteria are present that are actively causing an infection is treatment required. There are dozens, if not hundreds of "Strep" strains. The only strain that is tested for when throat problems arise is GABHS, or Group A Beta-Hemolytic Streptococcal bacteria, as this particular strain has been found to potentially cause kidney and heart disease. Antibiotics are both useful and necessary when symptoms such as enlarged tonsils with obvious pus, high fever and swollen neck glands exist. But what I find is that one of the most common reasons to give an oral antibiotic is throat pain, with no other evidence of infection whatsoever. The same situation applies to ear pain as well.

The more important question to ask is: What else could be causing the throat pain? The two most common reasons are allergies and acid reflux. Chronic post-nasal drip from the nose for any reason can cause throat irritation, producing symptoms from a slight tickle or irritation to pain. Hoarseness with or without a cough may also be present.

Acid reflux of the throat (called laryngopharyngeal reflux disease, or LPRD) is probably one of the most underdiagnosed conditions affecting the throat and can mimic allergy, cold and sinusitis symptoms. Despite extensive descriptions in basic medical texts and the lay press, physicians and patients are often too focused on gastroesophageal reflux disease (or GERD). For whatever reason, acid can come up silently into the throat and irritate the throat structures, causing or aggravating any of the following: throat pain, throat clearing, hoarseness, lump sensation, difficultly swallowing, tightness, burning, post-nasal drip and chronic cough.

You may be asking why acid comes up to the throat in the first place. There are a number of proposed reasons, too many to mention, but let's go back to one process that's related to the paradigm. If the tongue falls back and you try to inhale against a closed throat, a very high vacuum pressure is created in the chest, which overpowers the sphincter that closes off the stomach from the lower esophagus. The more acid there is hanging around in the esophagus, the more likely it can leak up through the upper esophageal sphincter (which separates the upper esophagus from the throat and is located behind the voice-box). This process results in irritation of the throat. Acid then causes more swelling in the throat, aggravating further tongue collapse, thus perpetuating the impaired sleep-breathing cycle.

As noted in previous chapters, acid that is present in the throat can end up in either of two locations:

1. It can descend into the windpipe. There are numerous studies showing that pepsin, a stomach enzyme, can be used as a marker of stomach acid traveling into the lungs. The inhalation of any liquid sitting in the throat is called aspiration. If this happens on a massive scale, such as in a hospital setting after

an operation, pneumonia can result. But most people have experienced a minor version of this phenomenon when a small amount of stomach acid reaches the throat. The feeling is very intense, with severe burning triggering the need to cough. But imagine if this was happening on a low-grade chronic level, where microscopic amounts of stomach juices leak slowly into the lungs. The stomach contains many substances that are irritating to throat or lung tissues such as acidic or alkaline material, digestive enzymes, food particles, and even bacteria. While the stomach and the esophagus are designed to effectively deal with this material, the delicate areas of the throat and lungs are not, and so problems result.

2. It can ascend into the ears, nose and sinuses. It's been proven in multiple studies that acid, pepsin, and *H. pylori*, a common bacterium found in the stomach that can cause ulcers, can travel into the sinuses and ears. Remember the last time you were drinking milk and you laughed, causing the milk to go up into your nose? Imagine doing the same with orange juice, and lastly, with vinegar. Imagine this process continuously happening on a microscopic scale when you are sleeping.

When you are lying down in bed and acid is drawn up from the stomach to the throat, it has a direct line to the back of your nose (the nasopharynx). The Eustachian tube openings, the tubes that connect the nose to the ears, are located on either side of this area. They open slightly by the tugging action of your palatal and jaw muscles, especially when you swallow or yawn, equalizing pressure between the ears and nose.

When chronic acid irritation occurs, swelling ensues around the Eustachian tube opening, preventing proper pressure equalization. The same thing can occur when you fly in an airplane, because until you swallow, there is a relative pressure difference between the middle ear cavity (which connects via the Eustachian tube to your nose) and the outer ear canal, preventing proper vibration of the ear drum. This leads to a feeling of fullness or mild hearing loss, until you swallow. But if there's swelling in your nose, the pressure can't equalize, and your ears feel stuffy and can even be painful.

Sleep position can also influence which side of the head is affected by nasal or sinus problems. More often than not, whenever a patient comes in complaining of a one-sided ear fullness and pain, it is usually the same side that they prefer to sleep on. Chronic Eustachian tube congestion can lead to fluid accumulation and ultimately an infection in the middle ear cavity. If the sinus passageways are blocked as well, sinus headaches and sinus pain also result.

People with tongue collapse naturally like to sleep on their side or stomach. These positions keep the tongue from falling back especially during deeper sleep, when there is increased muscle relaxation. But for some people, this is not sufficient. They begin to have more frequent obstructions and arousals, especially when there is any kind of inflammation accompanied by swelling in the throat as a result of colds, allergies, weight gain, and even stress.

This explanation demonstrates why many people report that their "cold" started with a scratchy throat, then traveled up into the back of the nose, followed by ear fullness and pain. Nasal congestion and sinus backup may also result, which leads to sinus pressure and headaches, and possible chronic sinusitis that lingers for weeks or months.

The post-nasal drip that one typically experiences due to either infections or allergies is the result of mucous glands in the throat attempting to dilute the refluxed acid. In some cases there is no significant nasal discharge or even nasal congestion. But in most cases, patients almost always complain of either a runny or stuffy nose. This could well result from microscopic portions of stomach acid irritating the nose.

Another major reason why your nose may be stuffy or runny is from the sleep-breathing dilemma. As stated previously, frequent arousals lead to a low-grade chronic stress response which causes an imbalance of the involuntary nervous system. In people with throat acid reflux, this relative imbalance was found to be present. Any relative weakness of this portion of the nervous system causes the blood vessels inside the nose to swell up, causing congestion and a runny nose. This is called chronic rhinitis, or non-allergic rhinitis, as opposed to allergic rhinitis. Allergic rhinitis refers to a typical nasal allergy condition where the nose is overly sensitive to pollens, dust, pet dander, etc.

Non-allergic or chronic rhinitis patients are overly sensitive to pressure, humidity, or temperature changes. They can also be sensitive to perfumes, smoke, and other odors. It is possible to have allergic rhinitis, non-allergic rhinitis, or both. Either way, any degree of nasal congestion from any reason can cause a mild vacuum effect downstream, aggravating potential tongue or palate collapse, continuing the vicious cycle.

One interesting phenomenon that I see quite frequently is that whenever patients are given the antibiotic azithromycin for their sinus or throat "infections," many people feel much better. Sometimes they swear by it. However, in theory, this particular type of antibiotic is relatively useless for some types of bacteria because of a high incidence of resistance. There are a few possible explanations for their perceived feelings of well-being. First, it could be a placebo effect, whereby the mere fact that a doctor prescribed a pill leads to the patient feeling better. Improvement would have occurred whether or not the pill had an active ingredient or was comprised of sugar only. Another possible explanation is that whatever was causing the irritation spontaneously disappeared.

Lastly, there are numerous reports that azithromycin and other antibiotics of its class exhibit anti-inflammatory properties. This could occur because this class of medications stimulates muscles in the stomach so that it empties faster. So the less acid that's present in the stomach, the less chance there is for it to be forced up into the throat, with less inflammation and swelling and less potential for tongue collapse. Furthermore, for people who make too much acid in their stomachs due to H. pylori bacteria, a course of azithromycin can temporarily suppress the bacteria and lessen acid production.

One final issue that deserves mention is the recent finding that most cases of self-reported sinus pain and headaches are in reality a variation of a migraine attack of the sinuses.[1] Migraine attacks result in nerve ending irritation and nasal passageway swelling, which blocks sinus passageways, leading to sinus pressure and ultimately to infection. Regardless of whether nasal irritation is caused by allergies, colds, acid reflux, or a migraine attack, the end result is swelling of the sinus passageways. This can lead to nasal congestion, which can ultimately influence tongue collapse in susceptible people.

A variation of this phenomenon called Schluder's neuralgia may occur due to a deviated nasal septum (or spur), or narrowing of the sinus passageways. This can aggravate neurologic headaches as the presence of a bony protrusion pressing on sensitive nerve endings can aggravate neurologic headaches. Any degree of mucous membrane or turbinate swelling will push the swollen membranes into the bony spur, which can press on a nerve ending. Here, the whole side of the face and the sinuses become painful, and further swelling occurs in the sinuses, leading to a pressure buildup and ultimately an infection.

So the next time you have a typical cold or sinus infection, or if you suffer from lingering or recurrent colds, looking at it from a sleep-breathing viewpoint may help you to better understand and manage these conditions.

7 Prone to Panic Attacks, Depression & Anxiety

Julie is 32 years old and came to see me for chronic sinus pressure and ear fullness. She was fine until about two years ago when she slowly began to feel anxious. Her medical doctor prescribed an anti-anxiety medication, which helped somewhat, but not completely. She would over-react to any little stress, and was especially anxious during her periods. She noted she gained about 10 pounds in the past few years, and she's been increasingly tired, has trouble sleeping, and now has to take naps. Her father snores and has heart disease.

APART FROM EAR, NOSE AND THROAT PROBLEMS, two of the most common conditions that I encounter in my practice are depression and anxiety. While patients don't come to see me for my expertise in this area, I've noticed that a higher than normal number of people with routine chronic sinus or throat problems tend to have depression, anxiety, or both.

It's traditionally taught that poor sleep can be a symptom of chronic sinusitis, and this has been largely taken as fact. Our assumption so far is that if you have a condition such as a chronic sinus pain, the resulting discomfort will interfere with your sleep, leading to fatigue, mood problems and irritability during the day. This makes perfect sense and this logic can be applied to almost any medical ailment, including cancer or viral infections. In Julie's case, most physicians will assume anxiety issues are unrelated to her sinus problems or poor sleep issues.

I won't go specifically into the details on the origins of depression and anxiety—there are volumes of books and articles, with vastly opposing opinions on where mood disturbances originate and how to treat them. I'll leave that to the mental health experts. I'm only going to address anxiety and depression from a sleep-breathing perspective, since this is what I see on a regular basis. What I am asking you to do here is to at least consider the possibility that poor quality sleep itself may be a significant aggravating factor, if not the initiator of certain mental health conditions.

Again, this brings up the chicken or the egg question: Does depression lead to poor sleep, or does poor sleep lead to depression? I think most people will agree with me that one can definitely aggravate the other, leading to a vicious cycle.

Regardless of what causes these disorders, we know that psychotherapy, cognitive behavioral therapy, and even antidepressant medications all help, to varying degrees. Let me add one more form of therapy that I have seen work, which is to improve the quality of breathing during sleep. I have seen countless people with various upper airway breathing problems improve significantly from a psychological aspect, simply by addressing their specific breathing problems with either medicine or surgery. For example, many people with deviated nasal septums who don't improve with medical therapy sleep much better with a simple septoplasty operation. As a result, they are much more refreshed when they wake up in the morning, and have more energy during the day. I never performed psychological profiles or questionnaires before and after surgery, but I'm willing to bet a lot of money that there will be significant improvements.

The same goes for children whose breathing passageways are enlarged by undergoing tonsillectomy and adenoidectomy. It's remarkable what the parents report in terms of their children's improvement in behavior, school performance, and speech-language development. There are numerous reports in the medical literature that support this observation.

The most dramatic improvements that I have encountered are after definitive treatment for OSA. Whether a person is treated with CPAP (continuous positive airway pressure), a mandibular advancement device, or with surgery, the results can be significant. Obviously, not all forms of treatment work or are tolerated by all patients, but many of the ones that do find benefit from any of these options can experience dramatic improvements in their energy level and quality of life in general. Again, psychological profiles are not performed before and after treatment, but if they were, I'm confident that there will be a significant improvement in depression and anxiety scores. Many of my patients have tapered down their depression or anxiety medications, and some have even stopped taking them altogether (obviously under supervision by their mental healthcare professional).

My point here is that for people with certain mental health conditions who also have sleep-breathing issues, addressing the breathing issues can potentially improve mental health problems as well. Yet, mental health patients are rarely screened for breathing problems. My paradigm suggests that a significant number of people with mental health issues will also have sleep-breathing issues. It just makes sense. If you can't breathe, especially at night when you are in deep sleep, then you won't sleep well. If you don't sleep well, you won't feel well during the day.

Generalized sleep deprivation or any degree of inefficient sleep can have a wide range of effects, including simple fatigue, poor concentration, and irritability. There is a continuum from the very subtle, such as forgetting about an appointment, to the very obvious, such as causing a car accident while dozing at the wheel. Even very small amounts of sleep deprivation have been shown to decrease memory scores and reaction times. This is a worrying situation since most Americans report that they are sleeping one to two hours less than their peers were fifty years ago. With the age of the internet, 24-hour news stations, cell phones and all the other stressful distractions of life, this is not surprising.

Of more concern is that on top of the usual sleep deprivation that Americans are regularly subjected to, their quality of sleep is even worse. Add to this the presence of any mental health condition, and sleep quality degenerates even further. Throw in additional stressful events, such as a divorce, traveling to five cities in a week for meetings, and sleep quality continues to go downhill. It's no wonder that mental health issues, particularly depression and anxiety, are so common in the United States and other developed countries.

If you thought this was bad enough, there's one more thing. Recall from the anatomy chapter the hypothesis (as corroborated by certain dentists) that human facial jaw bones are narrower than those of our recent ancestors due to a change in diet and bottle feeding. In addition, the ability of humans to talk created a situation whereby the voice box dropped lower in the neck, allowing the tongue to fall back relatively easily. This, coupled with smaller modern-day jaws, means there's less room for the tongue to sit, so it's more likely to fall back and obstruct the airway, especially when lying on the back and in deep sleep.

So what does all this have to do with depression and anxiety? Let's go back to our typical person, aged in her early twenties, with mild upper airway resistance syndrome. She normally sleeps on her side and wakes up refreshed. But in recent years, since starting law school, she has gained about five to ten pounds, and notices that she's more tired during the day than she used to be. Her ability to focus and concentrate is not what it used to be either. She finds law school stressful.

Now let's magically zoom in on her throat while she's sleeping. She normally has to sleep on her side to compensate for her tongue that keeps falling back and waking her up when she sleeps on her back. But now that she is a few pounds heavier, there is increased narrowing in her throat which initiates further collapse in deep sleep, even on her side. With each inhalation, especially in deep sleep, her tongue falls back slightly, but at a certain point, it falls back completely, occluding her breathing. She takes two to three more breaths against a closed throat, struggling to breathe. What happens next determines what kind of symptoms she will experience, as well as which medical condition she may be diagnosed with. There are three general scenarios:

1. Just after her tongue occludes her breathing, she wakes up to light sleep subconsciously and continues to sleep. This cycle happens repeatedly throughout the night. She will have various levels of arousal, some mild, and others she may be aware of. She used to have very vivid dreams, but now she doesn't dream as much. Regardless, the number of times she is aware of awakening is only the tip of the iceberg. Lack of continuous stable deep sleep can make her feel tired during the day. As a result, she may not be interested in undertaking her usual routine during daylight hours. Her focus and mental clarity may be diminished. She starts wondering why she's feeling this way and seeks the advice of the school psychologist. After undergoing some counseling, she starts taking an antidepressant and feels better, but never back to what she used to be. Thirty years later, she is diagnosed with OSA.

2. Just after her tongue occludes breathing, she takes two to three deep breaths against her closed throat, and suddenly wakes up violently, gasping for air, heart racing, and in a sweat (the fight or flight response). She is terrified, and feels that she is going to die. Of note, she wakes up while she's on her back. After a few minutes, she feels a little better. She rolls over to her usual left side, and goes back to sleep. This happens a few times every week. She also has frequent vivid dreams. During the day she feels a combination of mild fatigue and a state of uneasiness. At night, before she goes to sleep, she worries that these episodes may happen again, and has trouble sleeping. She naturally begins to worry about her finals the next day, and how she may fail if she doesn't get enough sleep. During the exam, she has a panic attack, but

gets herself together to finish and pass the exam. She also gets frequent stress-related headaches and neck spasms. Twenty years later, she is diagnosed with fibromyalgia.

3. Just after her tongue occludes her breathing, and after two to three inhalational breaths, she stops breathing completely for fifteen seconds. A few minutes later, she has another episode, but this time, the airflow into her lungs is only 20% of her normal intake, and this also lasts about fifteen seconds. Her oxygen level drops slightly during these episodes. These incidences occur, on average, fifteen times every hour during sleeping. She is diagnosed with OSA and does well with treatment.

The above three scenarios describe the same person with the same anatomy and life situations, but three different possible outcomes after her tongue occludes her breathing. What determines in which direction she follows is ultimately controlled by her involuntary nervous system. People with upper airway resistance syndrome have a nervous system that is intact, so any degree of impending obstruction is quickly sensed by the sensory nerve endings in the throat by the brain, and the order is given to wake up so that the muscles in the throat can tighten again, preventing continued collapse.

Waking up and disturbing the deep sleep phase is a good compromise for the alternative: stopping breathing completely. If you wake up suddenly and violently, then you are aware of these episodes, and depending on how your body reacts to this phenomenon, you will have different symptoms. Some patients report that they wake up on their backs, feeling like they were suffocating or choking. If you wake up to light sleep subconsciously, you won't be aware of interrupted breathing, but will be puzzled as to why you're so tired all the time.

People with OSA are thought to have diminished responses to impending airway collapse. This is why they are prone to long breathing pauses. Over time, these breathing pauses cause a tremendous vacuum effect upstream, causing the soft palate and the surrounding throat tissues to collapse, aggravating snoring. With repeated obstruction and desensitization of these nerve receptors, UARS patients frequently progress to OSA in later life.

There are six criteria that must be met for a clinical diagnosis of generalized anxiety disorder (GAD). It's interesting to note that one of these six criteria includes the six symptoms listed below. Of these six symptoms, a person needs to display three or more of the following for a period of at least 6 months:

- Restlessness or feeling keyed up or on edge
- Being easily fatigued
- Difficulty concentrating or mind going blank
- Irritability
- Muscle tension
- Sleep disturbance (difficulty falling or staying asleep, or restless unsatisfying sleep).

Notice how the symptoms that arise as a result of the case scenario that I described match to the letter the above diagnostic criteria. Granted any of these six symptoms or other forms of anxiety can be associated with many other medical or psychological conditions, but the point here is that the sleep-breathing paradigm could potentially lead to many of the symptoms associated with anxiety or depression.

I recently read a poignant article describing one person's experiences with panic disorder.[1] Although this differs from generalized anxiety disorder, he did mention in his article that his attacks occurred frequently at the end of dreamless naps. This is significant because the tongue is most likely to collapse during deep sleep, especially when on your back. More importantly, he wrote this article about his initial experiences as a college student in the 1970s. His panic disorder did improve, but continued to bother him for years. Interestingly, he came to see me over thirty-five years after his initial bout of panic disorder seeking treatment for his recently diagnosed OSA.

Another excellent example is a case report from 1998 where a Vietnam War veteran with post-traumatic stress disorder had complete resolution of his condition just after treatment for his newly diagnosed OSA.[2]

Most cases of panic disorder, depression, schizophrenia, bipolar disorder and obsessive-compulsive disorder begin in early adulthood. It's no coincidence that early adulthood is when our facial bones are fully developed (or under-developed), and our voice boxes are fully descended. Although the female voice box does not descend to the same extent as males, their jaws are slightly more recessed compared to men. This could also explain the higher incidence of "light" sleepers and cold hands in women. It is also is a good mechanical explanation of how the proposed maternal protection process works. This paradigm predicts that these issues are mainly a human phenomenon, and that with a few exceptions, there is significantly less depression or anxiety problems in the non-human animal kingdom.

There's a lot of controversy as to what causes panics attacks, depression and anxiety. Some feel that it's mainly a cognitive, mis-information-driven result, whereas the other extreme espouses a biochemical explanation. There are elements of truth to both theories. But consider the possibility that a sleep-breathing problem can alter both your cognitive state, as well as your brain biochemistry.

I'm not saying that all people with depression and anxiety disorders have a sleep-breathing problem. But based on the implications of what I have described in this book, it's even more important to ask about sleep issues if you have anxiety or depression. This is important especially if you are young, thin, female, a non-snorer, or otherwise don't fit the typical OSA stereotype. It's possible that by treating the sleep-breathing condition first, you may be able to avoid life-long counseling sessions, and harmful medications as well.

8   Men, Hot Flashes & Night Sweats

John is a 24 year old man who suffers from chronic nasal congestion. He took two courses of oral antibiotics for sinus infections in the past 6 months. After changing to a new job that's more sedentary, he gained about 10 pounds. He complains of daytime fatigue, and waking up in the middle of the night drenched in sweat. During the day, he feels too hot or too cold, and sometimes he breaks out in a cold sweat. He notices that he's been more irritable lately and feels like he's on edge all the time. His mother is overweight, snores "like a chainsaw" and is on medications for high blood pressure, diabetes and high cholesterol.

ABOUT ONCE EVERY MONTH, for the past few years, I've noticed an unusual pattern develop amongst some of my young male patients. The reason I had not noticed it until recently was because the details came to me in disjointed fragments, like many pieces of a complex puzzle. This remained the case until I began putting the pieces together in a whole new way. Once I did, a picture began to emerge of a typical young man in his early twenties, complaining of the common symptoms of menopause.

You're probably puzzled by my statement about men having menopausal symptoms. But let me explain. I would occasionally see young men who came to see me for routine sinus infections, complain of other symptoms such as: chronic fatigue, mood-swings, irritability, insomnia, poor sleep, night sweats, hot flashes, and weight gain. At first, I was puzzled too, since these were obvious signs of menopause in women that were happening in men. But what ultimately solved the puzzle was the fact that all these young men were eventually diagnosed with OSA. Later, I realized that middle aged women did not have a monopoly on these symptoms—all age groups of both sexes were just as prone, only not nearly so much as menopausal women.

Before I explain the answer to this mystery, let's go over some basic fundamentals of menopause as it relates to sleep-breathing problems. It goes without saying that women have issues related to reproductive physiology that vastly differ from men. As you may know, menopause is a natural process in which women slowly lose estrogen and progesterone production over years in their mid-life as their reproductive functions slowly diminish. As this process unfolds many women undergo some dramatic changes. For one thing, with decreasing estrogen and progesterone levels, women's rate of cardiovascular complications increase. In fact, by the time women are past menopausal age, their incidence of heart disease rises dramatically, almost catching up with that of men. One of the many explanations for this is that female hormones may protect women from heart disease. Another change that occurs at this time is that post-menopausal women tend to gain weight. Again, the theory is that the fluctuating hormone levels (especially lowered thyroid levels) decrease their metabolism and as a result make them more susceptible to weight gain.

What I believe to be the change that trumps all others listed above is that, during the transitional phase of menopause, women begin to experience loss of protective upper airway reflexes that are associated with the former high estrogen and progesterone levels of pre-menopause. As a result, if these women already had narrow airways to begin with, they are more likely to experience partial or complete muscle relaxation during deep sleep, since this is when muscles relax the most. Tongue muscle relaxation results in partial or total upper airway obstruction, causing you to wake up many times, preventing quality deep sleep. This process can lead to fatigue, night sweats, hot flashes, mood swings and irritability. Those few extra pounds that most women gain during menopause also serve to narrow the throat further, exacerbating the problem.

The narrower the airway, the more severe the symptoms that women may experience while undergoing menopause. This could be an important reason why different women progress through menopause with varying degrees of distress: Some have severe symptoms whereas others have minimal to no problems whatsoever.

But again, why are young men in their early twenties, who don't undergo such hormonal fluctuations, still experiencing the very same symptoms that women in their fifties experience at menopause? The connection between the two lies in how well they breathe while sleeping at night.

Poor sleep quality and fatigue are two of the most common complaints of menopausal women. One of the prominent theories that attempts to explain menopausal symptoms from a global perspective is that fluctuating levels of estrogen somehow affects the circadian rhythm patterns in the brain, leading to poor sleep.

Hot flashes and night sweats are common in menopause, but these events are also known to occur with any sudden hormonal level changes such as after hysterectomy, breast cancer chemotherapy, or even withdrawal from testosterone-blocking medications for men with prostate cancer. Both men and women can suffer from these common involuntary nervous system reactions. These symptoms are usually blamed for frequent arousals and poor quality sleep, but observed from the sleep-breathing paradigm, the hot flashes and night sweats can also result from inefficient sleep due to obstruction and frequent arousals. It's interesting to note that the incidence of depression, obesity, hypothyroidism and high blood pressure increases during the menopause years. Not too surprisingly, the incidence of sleep-breathing problems (namely, OSA) increases significantly as well.

Basically, most men do not experience the massive hormonal changes that women do as they age, although this theory has recently been challenged. As a result, however, most men also miss out on the many added benefits that female hormones like estrogen and progesterone provide. An important benefit is that these two hormones tend to protect women's airways from collapse by promoting increased tongue muscle tone. Historically, medical science has shown that when estrogen is administered to men it can lower the severity of OSA, as well as the incidence of heart disease.

Along these lines, a recent study revealed that tongue muscle activity during wakefulness was much lower in post-menopausal women compared with pre-menopausal women.[1] Eight post-menopausal women were given conventional hormone replacement, and their tongue muscle activity increased significantly. The study concluded that estrogen and progesterone are thought to play a synergistic role in maintaining upper airway openness and muscle tone. It's been shown in other studies that it's predominantly progesterone that stimulates both respiration and increased tongue muscle tone.

Looking at this phenomenon on the sleep-breathing continuum line, this explains why some of my male patients complain of typical menopause symptoms. Let's say that you have a narrowed jaw combined with a potentially collapsible tongue, the latter can drop to the back of the oral cavity and occlude breathing, especially when sleeping on your back and in deep sleep. Normally you compensate by sleeping on your side or stomach, but every time you catch a simple cold, it seems to last for weeks. Furthermore, if you gain five to ten pounds, you'll feel more tired, and therefore more moody and irritable. Some people, while they undergo this relative "change" in their lives, whether it's from a cold, an allergy attack, mild weight gain or a major life stress, find that their involuntary nervous system goes into overdrive to compensate for the changes the body is undergoing. In other words, you experience hot flashes, fatigue, mood swings, and irritability, which are generalized nervous system reactions that either sex can experience.

This same principle can be applied to younger women who suffer from pre-menstrual syndrome, or PMS. Menopause can be thought of as a prolonged change in a woman's hormonal status, whereas a woman's monthly periods comprise normal cyclical hormonal fluctuations. Temporary changes in hormonal levels result in the same processes (slight weight gain, loss of airway protective reflexes, more frequent sleep arousals) which may lead to the typical symptoms of PMS (bloating, weight gain, mood swings, irritability, poor sleep, fatigue, headache, poor focus or concentration).

This explanation of menopause and PMS is not meant to be an exhaustive overview of the subject. Instead, it proposes an alternative viewpoint, asking you to look at both of these conditions from sleep-breathing perspective that's common to both men and women. The terms "menopause" or "PMS" have traditionally been assigned to women. But since men don't experience menses, perhaps a new name should be considered exclusively for men who suffer from these same symptoms. The sleep-breathing paradigm opens up new treatment options for both men and women who suffer from these common symptoms.

9 Sleep Position & Sex

Liz and Adam are engaged to be married in four months. They consulted me regarding Adam's chronic snoring in an attempt to iron out this problem prior to getting married. Adam normally sleeps on his side, but whenever he turns to his back, his snoring is intense. Occasionally they must sleep separately.

A N INTERESTING NEW TREND was reported in *The New York Times* about couples building new homes with two master bedrooms.[1] There were various reasons mentioned including different work schedules, crying children, late night e-mails, or going to the gym at 5:30 in the morning. But one of the most common reasons given was due to snoring.

Simply put, sleeping in separate bedrooms is not good for relationships. Obviously, snoring alone does not break up relationships, but if there are other areas of conflict, a snoring bed-partner or spouse can definitely aggravate an already tenuous situation.

Snorers typically snore more while sleeping on their backs. The sleepless bed-partner elbows the snorer in the ribs, prompting the snorer to wake up slightly and turn over, consciously or subconsciously, thus lessening the degree of snoring. This is what's known as the "bruised rib syndrome."

Various relationship theories about sleep position speculate that this side position, facing away from your bed-partner, is a sign of detachment. But from a more practical standpoint, it allows the bed-partner to sleep, and the snorer may sleep better as well, since there is potentially less tongue collapse in the side position. Regardless, a severe snorer will most likely have some degree of OSA, and OSA can potentially lead to depression, mood swings, irritability and loss of intimate desires. In essence, it can be argued that lack of intimate desires is the outcome of poor breathing while sleeping.

More often than not, the non-snoring sufferer is frequently a "light" sleeper, and wakes up to even the slightest sound, movement or light. It's not uncommon for each of the couple to have variations of a sleep-breathing condition. In some cases, the woman has UARS, which automatically heightens the person's involuntary nervous system and sensory forms of input. Ear plug marketers target their advertising towards people in this situation. If you've been kept up all night long because of your spouse's snoring, then I'd bet that you will be cranky and not "in the mood" the following day.

Chances are, the snorer is more likely to toss and turn, taking up lots of space in bed, and for some people, their limbs can flail or jerk around during sleep. Other poor sleep hygiene habits, such as watching TV in bed, eating late, exercising before bedtime, or getting to bed too late, exacerbate the problem. In addition to your spouse's continual snoring, you may also have a very stressful job, or other personal problems, and for these reasons you've had more trouble falling asleep, and often finding yourself waking up frequently during the night. A snoring partner will only add to your total stress load.

Whether you are the snorer or the snoree, physiologically, due to lack of sleep efficiency, your stress levels increase, subtly stimulating the "fight or flight" mechanism of the involuntary nervous system. As you may recall from Chapter 5 (Creativity, Stress & Breathing), there are certain organs and parts of the body (gastro-intestinal system, reproductive organs, skin, extremities) that are considered low priority when you are under stress. Suffice it to say, reproduction is not a high priority when you're being chased by a tiger. In this situation, the nervous system clamps down on the blood vessels which supply the sexual organs, diverting energy to where you really need it to fight the upcoming calamity. Hence heart rate and blood pressure increases, and blood is diverted towards the lungs, brain and major muscle groups, such as the legs.

For men, sexual arousal is controlled by the parasympathetic, or relaxation part of the involuntary nervous system, whereas orgasm is controlled by the sympathetic, or "fight or flight" aspect of the involuntary nervous system. You can imagine that if chronic low-grade stress exists due to a sleep-breathing problem, the sympathetic part dominates, preventing proper activation of the parasympathetic responses during sexual intimacy. It's no coincidence that the incidence of both erectile dysfunction (ED) and sleep-breathing disorders increases proportionately with age. Erectile dysfunction is thought to be a direct complication of common cardiovascular conditions (high blood pressure, high cholesterol, diabetes, heart disease) that are widespread in older age groups. The sleep-breathing paradigm suggests that ED is a direct consequence of what causes cardiovascular conditions, rather than a result of the cardiovascular conditions themselves.

For women, a similar situation takes place, whereby chronic low-grade stress responses lower sexual interest and drive. If the woman has UARS, she is also likely to have temporomandibular joint disease (dental grinding or clenching of teeth), migraine or tension headaches. In this situation, if she says, "I have a headache," she's telling the truth.

A natural corollary of the above process can be applied to infertility issues as well. Besides obvious anatomic problems, many couples undergo an intensive battery of tests, which usually all come back as normal. They just can't conceive, or the woman just can't maintain the pregnancy. If a significant amount of blood is constantly being shunted or diverted from your reproductive organs, this prevents optimal blood flow, lowering optimal functioning. Frequently, the woman must be placed on hormonal "overdrive" for pregnancy to take place. Add the stress of going through this entire grueling in vitro fertilization (IVF) process, wondering if and when you're going to conceive, and it's easy to see how the stress of infertility feeds back into the stress of improper sleep and the entire cycle repeats itself to the detriment of both partners.

An interesting example is a patient of mine with mild upper airway resistance syndrome who was going through the stressful process of IVF, but was unable to conceive. She focused so much of her time and energy on this process that she was eventually fired from her job. When she arrived for the fertility treatment the next day, her doctor asked her curiously, "Why are you in jeans? You're normally in business attire." She relayed that she had been fired. The doctor smiled, and said, "That's it! You're going to get pregnant." Sure enough, she did.

Come to think of it, with the theoretical rise in sleep-breathing disorders in America, it's probably not a bad idea for spouses to sleep separately, at least in the short term, while the root of the problem is being addressed. Snoring and frequent sleep arousals are potent signs, not only of dysfunctional breathing, but of long-term health problems in the future. Addressing the issue of snoring, upper airway resistance syndrome, or OSA with your doctor will not only improve your sex life but increase your overall health and vitality levels. Acting now to address sleep-breathing disorders may interrupt life in the short term but the long-term benefits are definitely worthwhile.

10 A Stimulating Discussion About ADHD

Peter is in college and has been taking Ritalin for years. He's always struggled in school, but with hard work, he made it to college. In his freshman year he gained 15 pounds, and has commenced snoring. He normally must sleep on his stomach, and never wakes up refreshed. At age 5, his doctor told him that he would grow out of his large tonsils. His father also snores and suffered from a heart attack at age 49.

MY SON JONAS USED TO SNORE HEAVILY from the age of about three, and by age five, he became increasingly tired at the end of each day. He couldn't focus or concentrate as well as he had when he was younger. I happened to look inside his mouth and not unexpectedly, his tonsils were very large. They were almost touching in the middle (referred to as "kissing" tonsils). My wife and I took him to a colleague who ended up performing a tonsillectomy and adenoidectomy. After a few weeks, we were amazed at the difference in our son. I had many patients tell me in the past what a big difference a tonsillectomy made to their child's behavior and well being, but it didn't hit home until I experienced it for myself.

Jonas simply slept much better, was more energetic during the day, and his behavior improved as well.

Tonsillectomy (with or without adenoidectomy) is one of the most common surgical procedures performed in the US. From the 1950s to the 1970s, it was almost a rite of passage to have your tonsils taken out by a certain age. At that time, if you had tonsils, they needed to be taken out. Thankfully, over the past few decades, the removal rate has dropped significantly once it was realized that many unnecessary surgeries were being performed.

In the 21st century, tonsils are taken out for one of two reasons only: chronic or recurrent infections, or sleep-breathing problems. Children with severe OSA have a classic appearance: They are mouth breathers with stuffy noses, their lower jaw is narrow, and the roof of the hard palate is arched up like a steeple, rather than relatively flat like a ceiling. It's important to note that there is wide spectrum of presentations in people with OSA—many may appear anatomically normal.

ADHD or attention deficit hyperactivity disorder is a well-documented, but controversial condition that presents in adults as well as in children. Symptoms include inattention, poor ability to focus or concentrate, poor memory, and periods of hyperactivity. There are many different variations of this condition. Depending on the study, it's thought that anywhere from 2–4% of American adults and as high as 10% of children may have this condition. This is five to ten times higher than in other countries. There are also significant variations between different regions in the US. Finally, boys are more commonly affected than girls.

There are many proposed reasons for why ADHD occurs, but it's generally thought of as a psychological or neurological disorder. Various studies have shown possible abnormalities of brain function or metabolism. There appears to be a genetic component as well. Treatment involves psychotherapy with or without medication. Alarmingly, the rate of children (and now adults) being placed on medications is climbing rapidly. In general, these medications are stimulants, and they tend to work very well.

The question you may ask then, is how can a stimulant medication make a hyperactive child normal again? The answer is obvious: The child is sleepy. While an adult becomes drowsy and lethargic when sleep deprived, children become jittery and can't sit still. A stimulant, by making a child less sleepy, allows for better focus and improved attention. While appearing to address the symptoms of ADHD, to prescribe a stimulant medication may only cover up the symptoms without addressing the cause.

Among the plethora of the papers, articles and commentary on ADHD, rarely is there any mention of surgery as a potential option for treatment. But in recent years, a small number of studies strongly suggest that, for a significant number of children with ADHD, performing a tonsillectomy can produce improvements in the condition.

One study published in 2006[1] showed that one year after tonsillectomy and adenoidectomy, 50% of children diagnosed before surgery with ADHD no longer displayed symptoms. This study recruited 78 children scheduled for adeno-tonsillectomy and 27 control children undergoing other procedures. All the children were given a formal sleep study and a battery of behavioral, cognitive, and psychiatric tests. Before surgery, 28% of children in the adeno-tonsillectomy group (22 children) and 7% of control group (2 children) were found to have ADHD (as defined by the Diagnostic and Statistical Manual of Mental Disorders, 4th Edition). One year after surgery, half of the 22 children with ADHD who underwent surgery had persistent ADHD, which was no different from the rate of ADHD in the control children. Interestingly, before surgery 51% of the adeno-tonsillectomy group and 4% of the control group were found to have OSA. One year after surgery, only 12% in the adeno-tonsillectomy group while 13% in the control group were found to have OSA.

The above study only adds to the numerous papers that link ADHD and sleep related breathing disorders. Another large questionnaire-based study of over 3000 parents found sleep-disordered breathing occurred in about 25% of children. Those with sleep-disordered breathing were found to have significantly more daytime sleepiness, problem behaviors, hyperactivity, inattention and aggressiveness.[2] Another study comparing 28 children with OSA against 10 children with normal sleep patterns found that the former displayed significantly more behavioral problems, and lower scores on sustained attention and verbal ability.[3]

Yet another study compared 73 children in a general psychiatry clinic versus 70 children in a general pediatrics clinic.[4] The study found that habitual snoring was more frequent (33%) in children with ADHD. The author of this study suggested that sleep-related breathing disorders could be a cause of ADHD in some children. He further calculated that 81% of children with ADHD who also snored, or around 25% of all children with ADHD, could be treated effectively. The tonsillectomy study mentioned in the beginning of this chapter was a follow-up study to confirm these numbers. What that study showed was that about 50% of children with ADHD could be helped via adeno-tonsillectomy.

A further case report involving adults described three adult men with a history of ADHD and Ritalin usage.[5] These men were also found to suffer from OSA. Once treated for OSA, two of the three men were weaned from Ritalin. The participants who experienced mild OSA elected to address the condition using a combined regimen of weight loss and conservative management. There exists dozens of additional studies that link sleep-related breathing disorders to ADHD, asthma, chronic cough, school performance, behavioral problems, etc.

Numerous studies report that children with ADHD do poorly on cognitive tests, memory skills, and focus and concentration tasks. There are similar studies that find the same results in children with OSA. There are even reports of an association between bed-wetting in children and ADHD. Not surprisingly, there are many reports of an association between bed-wetting and OSA. Do you see a pattern? What's the common link?

Removing tonsils and adenoids improves ADHD in some children, but what about the remainder who show no improvement? In the chapter on anatomy, I described a hypothesis that proposes that during the past century, our facial structures have changed to the point where the jaw arches are more narrow with a resultant increase in crowding of teeth. This leaves less room for the tongue in the mouth cavity, which in turn makes the tongue more susceptible to collapse. Removal of the tonsils will help most children, but many still continue to have narrowed airways due their smaller jaw structures. There's even speculation that a small but significant number of children who do well after tonsillectomy will still go on to develop OSA later in life. I observe this frequently in my own practice.

The frustrating aspect about tonsillectomy is that although many tonsils are being removed unnecessarily, there is a proportion of children whose tonsils are not being removed when all symptoms point to the fact that the child would be better off without them. I have many pediatric patients who are classic mouth breathers, fidgety, perform poorly in school and experience recurrent upper respiratory infections and/or asthma. When I look inside their mouths, they frequently have kissing tonsils. The parents report loud snoring, with pauses in breathing and gasping for air. They continue to receive multiple medications without treating the obvious problem. Despite my recommendation for tonsillectomy, some parents (and some doctors) think that the child will eventually grow out of it.

One of the more common misconceptions about tonsils is that they eventually shrink. Yes, they do in normal situations, after peaking in size from ages three to five. However, when they are subject to constant irritation due to allergies or acid exposure in the throat (from sleep apnea), they often remain permanently swollen. Enlarged tonsils will aggravate further collapse and obstruction, promoting more acid to be vacuumed up into the throat, causing additional tonsil swelling.

Another misconception is that tonsils are vital for immune system purposes, so they should never be removed. Tonsils are theoretically involved with immunity, but when they are so big that breathing becomes chronically difficult at night, this latter issue outranks a theoretical concept. Fortunately, there are many other areas of lymphoid tissue that are actively involved in immune system development.

Of great concern is that even minor levels of obstruction in small children can have detrimental effects on health. Whereas adults are defined as having OSA if they stop breathing five to fifteen times every hour, in children, anything above once per hour is considered abnormal. If OSA occurs in a child during rapid brain and nervous system development, it could cause long-term harm. This concern was recently confirmed in ongoing research that shows that even after OSA is properly treated and the child is overall much improved, researchers can measure certain mental and behavioral indices which, even after treatment, never fully attain the levels of unaffected children. Though very subtle, this implies that there may be long-term neurologic harm.

You may ask how the sleep-breathing paradigm can explain the brain function differences and biochemical changes that are observed. It's not too far-fetched to acknowledge that it's possible that multiple breathing pauses while sleeping at night can have a profound effect on the cardiovascular system, hormonal system, or the nervous system.

Obviously, not all children (or adults) with ADHD have a sleep-related breathing disorder, but if the above estimates are correct, countless numbers of children are being needlessly medicated. The American Academy of Pediatrics published practice guidelines in 2002, which recommends screening all children for snoring. I was once told by a sleep researcher that all school-age children in Iceland are routinely screened for sleep apnea. Along with the current US obesity epidemic which serves to aggravate sleep apnea, there are many compelling reasons for the United States to do the same.

11 Sleep Better, Lose Weight

Barbara has been struggling with her weight almost her entire life. No matter how healthy she eats or how much she exercises, she can only lose ten pounds. She wants to lose another 25 pounds. Over the past few years, she's noticed that she's become more tired during the day. She frequently skips her workouts, due to being increasingly tired and not able to motivate herself to get to the gym.

DIETING SEEMS TO HAVE OVERTAKEN baseball as our national pastime. There are many proposed reasons for the obesity epidemic, including factors such as poor diet, lack of exercise, genes, and simply eating too much. But what does weight have to do with breathing? As you've probably guessed by now, weight and sleep-breathing problems are tightly intertwined.

Recent research studies reveal that lack of sleep, or just poor quality sleep, is linked to obesity. The less you sleep, the more your body alters normal body signaling messengers that then cause you to eat more or gain weight. Two of these messengers are leptin and cortisol. Leptin provides information about energy status to regulatory centers in the brain. Low levels of leptin are associated with increased hunger. Levels increase at night partly due to day-time meal ingestion. In sleep deprived people, leptin was found to drop significantly at night. Cortisol stimulates hunger and food intake in humans, and has been found to increase in response to experimental sleep deprivation. Chronic insomniacs display high cortisol levels.

It has been demonstrated in clinical trials that low levels of leptin are associated with high levels of cortisol (especially in the evening), and vice versa. Leptin tells the body when it has eaten sufficiently. So sleep deprivation, by lowering leptin, raises cortisol, causing you to eat more.

Ghrelin is another hormone produced in the stomach that rises before meals and drops after eating—it's leptin's counterpart.

In rats, sleep deprivation causes them to eat more, and starvation results in less sleep. As you can see, sleep and appetite are closely related. Another recent psychology article revealed that sleep deprived people prefer to eat foods high in fat. This explains why sleep deprived people crave junk food, and are more prone to weight gain.

Thyroid stimulating hormone, or TSH, is also found to be mark-edly affected by sleep deprivation due the lowering of thyrotropin-releasing hormone, or TRH. Since thyroid levels affect metabolism, this will affect your weight as well. Sleep loss is also found to raise blood sugar levels. In addition, cortisol is known to elevate sugar levels as well. As you can see there is a complex relationship between sleep and many of the hormonal signaling mechanisms of the human body. What I have just described is merely the tip of the iceberg.

So how does this fit into the sleep-breathing paradigm? If you are thin and have upper airway resistance syndrome, you may com-pensate by sleeping on your side or stomach, and staying active. But over the years, small changes occur as we age that slowly activates an unhealthy sleep-breathing cycle, which aggravates mild weight gain. Even a 3–5 pound upward shift can make an impressive dif-ference in sleep quality. Mild weight gain can enlarge the fat cells in your throat, and this causes the soft tissues of the throat to grow inwards, encroaching on your airway. This aggravates more palate or tongue collapse which causes more arousals or apneas. This causes inefficient sleep, which accelerates the entire metabolic response that was described earlier. As you gain more weight you begin to have more apneas, eventually leading to high blood pressure.

In this fast-paced, high-stress society, sleep is the first thing that is sacrificed when we're short of time. When we do actually sleep, we may sleep inefficiently as this book propounds. Add to this scenario our poor diet habits, along with less physical activity, and it's not surprising that well over 70% of adults in this country are considered overweight or obese.

I'd like to touch very briefly on diets. I want to stress not only how weight gain can aggravate sleep-breathing problems, but that sleep-breathing problems, if you're predisposed, can aggravate weight gain. This is another crucial hypothesis of the sleep-breathing paradigm.

What many of the diets also don't formally address is quality of sleep. Even when sleep is discussed, it is assumed that it centers around a simple lack thereof, or insomnia, rather than a sleep-breathing issue. By first addressing any sleep-breathing problems you may have, you will find that the weight loss program you are following becomes more effective.

My general recommendations on the subject of diets is to avoid any method that stresses too much of one food type, or cuts out too much of another. Eat a variety of whole foods, i.e. natural, unprocessed foods with no added chemicals, fertilizers or additives. In other words, the less processing, the better. It's not only how much you eat, but what you eat, at what time and how frequently, that's of equal importance.

Being Korean, it's almost second nature for me to think of foods that we eat as important as medicine, rather than thinking about food simply as a source of nutrition and energy. I still remember my mother touting over and over again the beneficial health properties of certain vegetables or fish.

One of the most popular television dramas from South Korea in recent memory details the life of an orphaned girl who overcame all odds by being accepted to a rigorous training program in the royal court's team of cooks in ancient Korea. Her competitors became jealous and eventually had her tortured for conspiring to kill the king and then she gets banished to a remote island. There, she trained to become a physician and later re-entered the royal court as a physician-in-training. After the king became ill, she used her talents in the healing properties of food, as well as her medicinal training, to save the king's life.

I mention this television show because what I remember most from watching this very long mini-series is the intricate accounts and details involved in how food is prepared, and for what reason. One unique concept I found very interesting is that certain foods should be prepared for certain individuals. Not all nutritious food is good for all people. Each person benefits from a diet tailor-made for them and them alone. In a similar way, what you may find is nutritious for some people may not be nutritious for you. Needless to say, this series was an incredible hit in many parts of the world, largely because of the important message it contained.

Another East Asian food concept is the Sumo wrestler's diet. Sumo wrestlers eat two big meals a day (about 5000 calories).[1] They exercise intensely during the day without eating any breakfast, which lowers their metabolism. Then they eat lunch followed by a nap. After eating a big dinner, they go to sleep immediately. This fools their bodies into thinking that they are starving, promoting long-term energy storage and fat production. It's not hard to see that this method of eating works, and it works well! This method of eating may also sound uncannily familiar to some readers and may provide insight into inexplicable weight gain where the diet is fundamentally sound.

Eating just before bedtime is probably the single most common habit that can aggravate the sleep-breathing problem described repeatedly throughout this book. If your tongue falls back occasionally and you obstruct, you will take a few breaths inwards against a closed throat, causing that vacuum effect that extracts the contents of the stomach up into the throat. If there is more stomach acid present because you just ate a meal, then there is more acid to be sucked up into your throat, which can then go on to irritate your throat and cause further swelling, and cause more airway collapse.

Most diet experts recommend that you eat many small meals (four to five) divided evenly throughout the course of the day. One healthy way of eating is to choose foods that possess a low glycemic index. The glycemic index is a measure of how quickly the sugar content of food is absorbed into the bloodstream. Foods such as non-wholemeal pasta and white rice can be processed and absorbed quickly, resulting in a rapid rise in blood sugar. Conversely, barley and soymilk have low glycemic indices, taking longer to be digested and releasing sugars at a steadier rate into the bloodstream. With low glycemic index foods, you won't feel as hungry soon after you eat as is common with high-glycemic foods.

The "volumetrics" diet is another popular and newer way of eating that focuses on choosing foods with a high fiber and fluid content. This approach to eating is based on the fact that when your stomach is full, you'll stop eating. Eating foods with a high fluid and volume content (such as fruits, vegetables, non-fat milk, soups, air-popped popcorn) will make you feel full faster. It also focuses on avoiding foods with a high energy density (ED), i.e the number of calories in a given food divided by its weight. So naturally, foods high in fat or sugar (such as cookies, fried foods, soda, chips, fatty meats) have more calories in a smaller amount of volume, and thus, a higher ED. For more information on proper nutrition and exercise, browse our Expert Interview series at www.sleepinterrupted.com.

The texture and degree of processed foods also affects oral health and consequently weight. Recall the study by Price in the anatomy chapter who showed that indigenous people who ate off the land had perfectly placed teeth with wide dental arches and little evidence of decay. However, after the introduction of Western, processed foods, cavities appeared and the jaws of successive generations became increasingly narrow with associated crowding of teeth. It's ironic that the most developed countries in the world have the most nutritionally malnourished people when observed from a jaw development standpoint.

On that note, whenever someone aged between twenty and fifty comes to see me and they have upper airway resistance syndrome or OSA, I always ask about whether or not their parents snore, and what kind of medical problems their parents experienced. Almost unfailingly, one or both parents who were born and raised in America, who ate a standard American diet (i.e., SAD) would not only snore loudly, but have one or many of the complications of OSA, such as obesity, hypertension, depression, heart disease, and others. In contrast, patients with parents who still lived in non-First World countries mostly reported that their parents were very healthy. The less developed the country, the healthier the status of the parents. I doubt they have any less stress than we do, but they probably eat less processed foods.

So why then do so many people who diet and exercise have such a hard time losing weight? I'm willing to bet that if you look closely at their sleep habits, either they don't sleep long enough or something keeps them from achieving deep efficient sleep, such as a sleep-breathing problem. Not too surprisingly, many patients who have sleep related breathing disorders and are overweight find it easier to lose weight once they are treated for their sleep-breathing condition. So the next time you begin your diet program, make sure you incorporate a good sleep hygiene program. The subject of sleep hygiene is discussed in a later chapter.

12 Pregnancy, Sleep & Breathing

Kim is in her eighth month of pregnancy. Besides all the excitement and nuisances that accompany being pregnant, her husband Jonathan began complaining about her recent onset of snoring. Her nose is chronically stuffy these days, and her doctor is monitoring her blood pressure, which was slightly elevated on her last visit.

I ALLUDED TO A LINK BETWEEN pregnancy and OSA at the beginning of this book. Let me go back and summarize what happened. After delivering our first child, Jonas, my wife, Kathy, was severely depressed for a full year. She was told she had post-partum depression, and that nothing could be done. After suffering through an agonizing year, she eventually felt better.

I never gave that much thought until we had our second son, Devin. For four months following the delivery, she was severely dizzy and light-headed, especially when she got up to move around. She had not gained as much weight with this pregnancy. Kathy's blood pressure was always on the low side, but now it was even lower. She saw a number of doctors, and even went to the emergency room when she began to have numbness in her right arm, to make sure she wasn't having a stroke. Eventually, she got over her ill health after about four months, but only after losing all her pregnancy weight.

During this time, I had been reading an interesting article on evolution and OSA, which implied that due to the voice box descending to facilitate speech and language development, all humans are susceptible to varying degrees to the occurrence of tongue collapse (see Chapter 2 on anatomy). About the same time, I was seeing many younger patients who complained of some or all the following symptoms: various chronic nasal or sinus conditions, chronic fatigue, poor sleep, insomnia, not being able to sleep on their backs, cold hands or feet, low blood pressure, light-headedness or dizziness, depression or irritable bowel syndrome. This constellation of symptoms was described previously as upper airway resistance syndrome (UARS). UARS is different from OSA in that apnea patients stop breathing for 10–30 seconds after airway obstruction, whereas UARS patients awaken immediately when they obstruct, preventing them from getting deep restful sleep. All these patients had one thing in common on physical examination: When sleeping on their backs, their tongues collapse, almost completely occluding their airway to only a few millimeters.

Many of these UARS patients report that their problem started after a very stressful life event, a very bad cold or infection, after gaining a few pounds, or as a result of pregnancy weight gain. All of a sudden, my wife's situation made sense. Pregnancy, by producing weight gain, had aggravated her UARS. Only after she lost all her pregnancy weight did she feel completely better again.

Women in their third trimester are miserable in general, not only due to having a baby growing inside their abdomens, but due to the general weight gain. This causes their breathing passageways to narrow, aggravating collapse in certain susceptible individuals. Even normal healthy adults with a common cold don't sleep well, tossing and turning all night, only to return to normal once the cold resolves. Due to nasal congestion, a vacuum effect is created downstream, aggravating tongue collapse. The same thing can happen in pregnant women. The latter frequently complain of stuffy noses, especially in the third trimester, when estrogen and progesterone can aggravate nasal congestion.

There are some women who never improve after they deliver their babies. They are not able to lose weight, feel chronically tired, and never really feel normal again. In this scenario, the vicious cycle continues, with fatigue and poor sleep leading to an inability to exercise properly, with the consequent weight gain aggravating poor sleep. In addition, it's been shown that poor sleep efficiency makes the body gain weight and encourages the sufferer to preferentially choose unhealthy foods (see Chapter 11, Sleep Better, Lose Weight).

There are many studies on OSA and its effects as pregnancy progresses. There are other papers that even suggest that OSA may play a role in preeclampsia, a dangerous condition in pregnancy where high blood pressure develops. Application of CPAP (continuous positive airway pressure), where gentle air pressure is passed through a mask on the nose, lowered the elevated blood pressure in most of the women in one study.[1] Interestingly, these women did not fit the criteria for OSA; rather, they had multiple arousals—around 10 per hour—thus fitting the criteria for UARS. The authors did not state that all women with preeclampsia undergo treatment for OSA, but physicians should at least think about the possibility of a sleep-related breathing disorder. In these situations, knowledge of the mother's parents' medical histories may be helpful, especially if the latter snore severely and have the typical complications of OSA, such as hypertension, depression, or heart disease.

Another study revealed that babies of women who snored during pregnancy had lower birth weights and lower Apgar scores at birth.[2] The Apgar score is a way of quickly assessing a newborn's physical condition to determine if there's a need for urgent or further medical care. Low Apgar scores are not unexpected in such cases, as snoring implies partially obstructed breathing, with potentially detrimental consequences to the unborn baby.

Lastly, pregnant women who slept less than six hours per night had longer labor and higher cesarean deliveries (4–5 times higher) than women who slept longer hours.[3]

These are some of the many examples of various situations in pregnancy that could be explained by a temporary sleep-breathing condition. The added weight, especially in the third trimester, can narrow the throat, causing tongue or throat collapse. Weight gain and obesity tend to narrow the area above the tongue, in the area of the oropharynx (from the soft palate to just above the back of the tongue). If you are already susceptible (meaning you have a predisposed anatomy), then even minor weight gain can bring on symptoms. Problems persist if you are unable to lose a significant part of your pregnancy weight after delivery.

One piece of good news is that due to the increased levels of estrogen and progesterone during pregnancy, the body has more of a tendency to keep the airways open, even when there are forces that promote tongue or throat collapse. But once the baby is delivered, the body is left with the added weight, but no elevated protective hormone levels. This explains why it is so important to return to your previous non-pregnant weight and follow a sensible diet and exercise regimen to achieve this goal.

13 An Awakening Encounter with Insomnia

Jennifer is a 25 year old lawyer who complains of many weeks of facial pain and sinus pressure. Recently, she's noticed she's having a hard time falling asleep due to thoughts about work. Even when she does fall asleep, she usually wakes up briefly about two hours later, which causes her to be more stressed. She tosses and turns all night and is awoken by any little sound, noise or movement. Her old job allowed her to come home early and eat at 7 P.M. but now she comes home round 9 P.M. After preparing and eating dinner, she goes to bed around 11 P.M.

ALL OF US HAVE EXPERIENCED INSOMNIA at least a few times in our lives. Before every major examination (SAT, Medical College Admission Test, otolaryngology board exams), I never slept for more than three hours. I went to bed nice and early, wanting to go to sleep, but it just didn't happen…until about three in the morning.

Insomnia comes in various forms, but the most common types are sleep onset insomnia and sleep maintenance insomnia. Sleep onset insomnia means that you can't fall asleep when you want to, and sleep maintenance insomnia is when you keep waking up after you've fallen asleep, or wake up much earlier than you desire. Periods of insomnia can be brief, or they may be chronic. It's estimated that 10% of people in this country have chronic insomnia, and about 25% have problems with sleep at some point in their lives. These are staggering numbers. It's estimated that about 100,000 motor vehicle accidents occur every year due to drowsiness. We know that the older you are, the more likely you are to develop insomnia. Sleep difficulties are also more common in women.

There are a number of explanations for insomnia. The more obvious ones are stress, anxiety and depression. Certain medications and caffeinated drinks can have stimulating effects. Alcohol may make you fall asleep faster, but lessens the quality of your sleep. There are a number of behavioral issues, such as watching TV late in bed, eating in bed, and exercising just before bedtime, that can prevent proper sleep onset. Certain medical problems, such as cancer or chronic pain, can cause or aggravate insomnia. Major life changes such as menopause, retirement, job changes or intense stress can bring on this condition as well.

Let's assume that you've addressed all the issues above, or you haven't experienced any of them. You also don't have a particularly stressful life. But you still keep waking up, or are unable to go to sleep. You've tried sleeping pills in the past with success, but you resist taking them because of the potential for addiction. What can you do?

As there are a number of good books on what causes insomnia, I won't go into conventional theories in detail. But what I wish to propose in this chapter is that there are a number of people with insomnia who have a variation of the very same sleep-breathing disorder that I describe in this book. Conventional teaching in academia stresses that insomnia is a completely separate condition from OSA or any other sleep-breathing problem. They believe that regardless of what the cause, the end result is a state of central nervous system hyper-arousal, perpetuated by cognitive or behavioral factors, and therefore not a sleep-breathing issue whatsoever.

However, over the years, I've noticed that many insomniacs don't like to sleep on their backs. Plus they tend to report that they wake up after one to two hours and are unable to fall back asleep easily. They may also wake up repeatedly every one or two hours, or they wake up in the early morning hours, particularly around 4–6 A.M. What's remarkable about these timeframes is that they mirror the cycles that normal sleep follows, from light to deep and from deep to light sleep. Most people go through three to five of these cycles per night, with progressively longer REM (or the dream state) stages near the end of the night. The time from sleep onset to the first REM state is about 90–120 minutes. Is it a coincidence that insomniacs wake up at the same first time interval? We also know that when people wake up too early (around the 4–6 A.M. mark), this coincides with the time that most people have the longest period of REM sleep. REM sleep is when all the muscles of your body, including your throat, relax. If your anatomy is predisposed to collapse and obstruction, then your tongue will fall back and cause you to wake up.

As one gets older, the soft tissues of the throat start to loosen and sag, and with each breath over time, either the tongue or the soft palate slowly stretches inwards. This is why most senior citizens with insomnia that I examine have a very small space in the back of the throat, behind the tongue. Healthy, vibrant senior citizens will usually have wide open throats with no significant tongue collapse. Coincidentally, both insomnia and sleep-breathing problems get worse as you get older.

In essence, one could argue that what's classically described as insomnia is really the onset of upper airway resistance syndrome (UARS). You may recall that UARS patients have very narrow oral cavities and their tongues tend to fall back and collapse easily, especially when they are on their backs and in deep or REM sleep. If tongue collapse with obstruction is present in young adults who have problems sleeping, then the person will most likely be diagnosed with UARS, but if these symptoms occur in a sixty-year-old patient, it's much more likely to be labeled insomnia.

There's also an observation that depression may be linked to insomnia. I would think that if you can't sleep properly, it's not surprising that you may feel depressed. One could also aggravate the other. This is another example of looking at individual trees without seeing the whole forest. We can do study after study looking at the relationship between these two conditions, but wouldn't you agree that if a sleep-breathing problem could explain both insomnia and depression, this would be a simpler, more satisfying explanation?

The only way to prove what I'm saying is to do studies on insomnia patients (using pressure catheters in the throat), to determine whether some degree of obstruction is present, especially when flat on their backs. The problem with sleep studies is that, in general, they are designed to pick up mostly apneas (greater than ten second pauses in breathing) and hypopneas (lesser versions of apneas). If you stop breathing for two to three seconds and then wake up to a light sleep or completely awaken, then it's not counted as an apnea. This could be happening 20–30 times every hour and you'd be told there's nothing wrong with you. As long as we hold onto certain accepted paradigms (that insomnia is unrelated to sleep-breathing problems), a study like this is unlikely to happen. There's even a running joke in the scientific community that the National Institutes of Health (NIH) will not fund a major study unless it's been done many times before.

I'm not disagreeing with any of the mainstream opinions on insomnia. There are countless important studies and findings that have shed invaluable light on this important topic. My point is that there may be some insomniacs who may respond to treatments that are designed more for sleep-breathing problems. One good example is when I tell patients with insomnia to avoid sleeping on their backs, in some instances, sleep quality improves.

Unfortunately, the main focus of the sleep medical community is on developing newer and better sleeping pills, trying to target that one brain receptor that will put you to sleep for exactly eight hours without causing any drowsiness or other side effects. Fortunately, great strides have been made in other non-pharmacologic forms of treatment such as cognitive behavioral therapy (CBT).

Before you even consider getting professional help, start with basic good sleep habits as outlined in Chapter 23. Try alternative or herbal remedies, such as melatonin or valerian. Educate yourself on this condition first, rather than relying on a sleeping pill. Whether via medications, alternative therapies, CBT, or perhaps the suggestions in his book relating to sleep-breathing problems, most people can be treated effectively for chronic insomnia.

14 Cold Hands, Warm Heart

Jessica is a 39 year old woman who suffers from monthly migraines related to her periods. She sleeps with mittens and socks on her hands and feet, no matter how warm the temperature. She is chronically tired, and never feels refreshed, even after sleeping for ten hours, usually on her stomach. She recently underwent testing for chronic diarrhea and bloating, and was told she may have irritable bowel syndrome.

THE WELL-KNOWN PROVERB, "cold hands, warm heart" is frequently used by mothers to reassure their daughters that having cold hands meant that they have a warm and caring heart. The original roots of this saying referred to certain cold and reserved people having kind hearts. For many women (and men), this may be literally true. There are millions of women and men who have excessively cold hands or feet, especially in colder climates. This condition, where one has cold or numb hands or feet, without any obvious medical cause, is called Raynaud's phenomenon. If it also involves one of many known autoimmune or other medical conditions, then it's called Raynaud's disease.

For most people it's not so bothersome, but for many, circulation can get so bad that the fingers or toes turn purple. Sufferers generally compensate by avoiding cold temperatures, but some must routinely wear mittens or socks on their hands and feet at night, even in the summer. If you've ever shaken hands with someone with this condition, you know what I'm describing. In fact, this person does not even have to have cold hands per se, but frequently self-perceives that their hands are cold.

Many years ago I noticed a pattern amongst my patients with chronic sinusitis or frequent migraine headaches. Most complained of cold hands. In addition, almost all stated that they preferred not to sleep on their backs. They all had various degrees of daytime fatigue, and they all had either a runny or stuffy nose. Most were young thin women (and men as well) who did not snore. Their blood pressures were reported to be normal or on the low side, and many of these people complained of dizziness and lightheadedness when they stood up too quickly.

When I went to the scientific literature, these various symptoms were very similar to a syndrome coined UARS, or upper airway resistance syndrome. As you may recall from the discussion on this topic from Chapter 3, people with UARS are generally thin women (and men) who are unable to obtain quality deep sleep due to frequent upper airway obstruction and arousals. The most common culprit is the tongue, which is anatomically predisposed to falling back, especially when sleeping on their backs, and when they reach deep sleep.

Let's review the sleep-breathing paradigm again. You naturally like to sleep on your side or stomach, but it doesn't completely prevent your tongue from falling back and obstructing, especially in deep sleep. Due to multiple arousals, you can't get deep efficient sleep. This causes a low-grade stress response which preferentially activates the stress (fight or flight) part of your involuntary nervous system. Sometimes you'll wake up suddenly, feeling like you were choking or suffocating, struggling for breath and your heart racing. If you think you're under attack all the time when you are sleeping, it's only natural that this feeling can carry over into the daytime as well.

For example, if you are suddenly being chased by a tiger, your first priority is to run away. In this situation, you need to mobilize all your energy and blood-flow to your central muscles, and to your heart and brain. If you think that you are constantly under attack all the time, then you won't digest well or have blood circulating in your hands or feet. This is why hands tend to feel colder when you are under stress. Sometimes the nervous system in the hands become confused and may get numb, sweaty or even too hot.

Besides cold hands and feet, people with UARS have various other symptoms, including low blood pressure, sinus headaches, migraines, TMJ, constipation, diarrhea, bloating, depression, anxiety, and fatigue. Whether the blood pressure is normal or low, many feel dizzy or lightheaded when they stand up too quickly. Depending on what the predominant symptom is, you could be given a particular diagnosis. If you have mainly severe long-term fatigue, then you may be given the diagnosis of CFS; for chronic pain, fibromyalgia; for chronic diarrhea, constipation, bloating, irritable bowel syndrome.

One very interesting historical note is that in the late 19th and early 20th centuries, there was a term called neurasthenia, used to describe women who suffered from an unexplainable host of symptoms such as chronic fatigue, weakness, chronic pains, dizziness, and passing out. Modern doctors now see this as an imbalance between the two opposing halves of the involuntary nervous system. More recently, neurasthenia has been renamed to dysautonomia. Typically, patients' symptoms are out of proportion to what was objectively seen. Doctors in this country use the term dysautonomia for severely debilitating cases, but in Japan, I am told that an involuntary or autonomic nervous system imbalance of even small degrees is considered significant.

This brings up an obvious question: Are dysautonomia and UARS describing the same condition? All the features and symptoms sound surprisingly similar. Both are aggravated by stress or simple viral illnesses. Both result in frequent or prolonged infections that linger or just never go away. Most people with both conditions find that eventually (years to decades later) it does fade away. The similarities are truly striking.

There are a number of explanations for UARS that explains its similarity to dysautonomia. One is that in UARS, constant arousals at night lead to a chronic stress state, confusing the involuntary nervous system, which leads to the general list of symptoms described above, with a few variations. You could say that the nervous system is hypersensitive or overactive to some degree.

Another explanation is the fact that viewed from the sleep-breathing paradigm, any process or event that promotes and accelerates the sleep-breathing problem can definitely aggravate a wave of major symptoms. This includes major stress, slight weight gain, or a simple cold or allergy attack. All these events can directly or indirectly promote swelling or narrowing of the upper airway, which self-perpetuates the vicious cycle.

I don't have any twenty to thirty year-long follow up studies on UARS patients, but a number of my original UARS patients have been found to have significant OSA three to five years after their original UARS diagnoses, especially if they have gained weight. Conversely, many of my middle-aged or older patients with OSA tell me that when they were younger, they were thin, had cold hands, low blood pressure, chronic diarrhea, or migraines but, with age, these symptoms have lessened, except for the fact they are now significantly more overweight, they snore, and they have high blood pressure.

Some UARS patients stay the same throughout their senior years, but in my experience, most tend to put on weight gradually in later years and progress into OSA. We know that in OSA patients, the autonomic nervous system responses are blunted, potentially explaining why they stop breathing for so long. Even their heart rates don't slow down like they normally do when they exhale (exhalation activates the parasympathetic or relaxation portion of the involuntary nervous system).

There are many other valid explanations for cold hands, but the sleep-breathing based explanation makes a lot of sense. A great example is one of my patients with severe UARS and mild OSA, whose cold hands got significantly better after definitive surgical management of her tongue collapse. Many of her other symptoms improved as well. The beauty of this paradigm is that it doesn't contradict any other theory or explanation in current mainstream thought.

Cold hands may mean a warm heart when you're young, but when you're older, having warm hands may signify a cold heart—where not enough blood flows to the heart after coronary artery disease sets in.

15 Sleep & the "C" Word

May is a 55 year old woman who has been suffering from recurrent sinus infections, chronic post-nasal drip and hoarseness. She complains of intense fatigue to the point of not being able to function at work, or spend quality time with her husband. Her life has been difficult ever since undergoing surgery and chemotherapy for breast cancer three years ago. She used to sleep on her stomach all her life, but was forced to sleep on her back since the operation due to the discomfort of the incision. As a younger woman, she was quite thin and used to have cold hands and feet, which improved over the years. She has slowly gained about twenty pounds over the past twenty years.

IT'S COMMONLY KNOWN THAT CANCER PATIENTS have trouble sleeping. There's no surprise as to why this is so. Either due to pain or the effects of treatment (surgery, radiation therapy or chemotherapy), cancer patients seldom sleep well. Just knowing that you have cancer can also keep you from sleeping well at night. But is it possible that poor sleep can lead to cancer?

It's generally acknowledged that lack of deep sleep may prevent proper immune system function, potentially leading to cancer. Countless other sources have stated or suggested that stress can lead to cancer as well. But what about improper breathing at night due to repeated obstruction, with arousals or apneas?

During my research into the sleep-breathing paradigm many years ago, I noticed an interesting similarity between findings in cancer research and cardiovascular disease research. Many of the cell-to-cell and cell-to-body signaling mechanisms were very similar, if not the same.

For example, vascular endothelial growth factor (VEGF) is a cellular signaling substance that promotes new blood vessel formation. It's essential to organ and tissue health, and is required when oxygen supply in the body is compromised. Prolonged breathing pauses seen in OSA can lower blood oxygen levels, leading to what is called hypoxia. Interestingly, VEGF was found to be elevated in OSA patients, but returned to normal levels after appropriate treatment.[1]

Similarly, there are a number of cancer research studies that show that VEGF plays a role in tumor growth. Hypoxia usually kills normal cells, but cancer cells can overcome this process by recruiting more blood vessel formation by producing higher levels of VEGF. As growing cancer cells begin to outstrip the blood supply, they need to promote new blood vessel growth so the cancer can receive more nutrients. Hypoxia has been shown to trigger a series of signaling processes in cancer cells that raise local tissue levels of VEGF. This process was reported to occur in human breast, uterine, cervix, bladder, liver and pancreatic cancers, where hypoxia was found to stimulate hypoxia inducible factor 1 (HIF-1), which promotes VEGF production.[2-4] Additionally, chronic hypoxia was demonstrated to cause genetic mutations in the p53 tumor suppressor gene, which is a common and well-studied gene in a variety of cancers.[5]

Furthermore, both cardiovascular disease and OSA are associated with elevations in c-reactive protein (CRP), interleukin-6 (IL-6), tumor necrosis factor, fibrinogen (a protein associated with clot formation), and other inflammatory markers.[6] The same markers of inflammation are also found to be elevated in certain cancers as well. There are tomes of studies in this area—I'm just scratching the surface.

If you have OSA, the resultant chronic hypoxia due to multiple breathing stoppages can lead to various physiologic events that promote cardiovascular disease. But even in lower degrees of sleep apnea or even UARS patients, there may be consequences via the following mechanism. By definition, people with UARS don't have hypoxia—they never stop breathing long enough to have significant hypoxia. But repeated short breathing pauses with multiple arousals can lead to a low-grade stress response, which preferentially activates your fight-or-flight response. This can shut down blood flow to "unnecessary" body parts and organs, such as your extremities, gastrointestinal system, and genito-urinary system. Chronically shutting down blood flow to these body parts and organs could then promote hypoxia, vascular recruitment, and abnormal tissue growth.

Interestingly, if you look at the 2007 cancer statistics from the American Cancer Society the top three new cancers diagnosed in women in descending order (excluding lung cancer) are breast, colon/rectum, and uterine cancer. In men the top three are prostate, colon/rectum and bladder. Notice that organs and structures that you need when you're under stress (heart, muscle and brain) are not in the top ten for either men or women. The top three areas for both men and women happen to be organs that are considered "low priority" when the body is under stress. Although I left out lung and bronchus (most of these cancers are due to smoking), and skin cancers (most are due to sun exposure), one could make the argument that less oxygen from apneas or arousals make these body areas more susceptible to cancer formation, especially if chronically irritated by smoking or sun exposure.

I realize this theory is a bit of a stretch, but looking at it as a whole, it doesn't contradict current cancer research findings. It may be a weak explanation when it comes to molecular and genetic models for cancer, but on a more holistic level, this may explain why almost every time I see a woman with a history of breast cancer, they almost always admit that they have cold hands, fatigue issues, and are unable to sleep on their backs, even years before the cancer diagnosis. Frequently, one of their parents had a severe snoring problem, or a history of heart disease.

We also know that the immune system is vital in preventing cancer cells from progressing; it's constantly on the lookout for mutations and early cancers, eradicating these cells before they begin to cause harm. If your immune system is not functioning optimally, and the body is chronically deprived of adequate oxygen levels or blood flow, then a cancer can hypothetically arise.

There are also many intermediate steps that can occur long before cancer develops. Constant stimulation of blood vessel and tissue growth by these "renegade" cells can cause local organ tissue enlargement, without it being a true cancer. Take, for example, breast fibrocystic disease, thyroid nodules, ovarian cysts, or prostate enlargement. If these organs are constantly deprived of blood due to hypoxia, certain mutated cells will generate factors that promote new vessel formation with local tissue enlargement. As these cells continue to grow, whether in an isolated area such as a nodule or cyst, or involve the entire gland, symptoms may arise such as urinary difficulty in men and the presence of a breast lump in women.

Some of these "benign" growths can turn into true cancers. This has been confirmed in findings that show that the rate of cancers in these benign growths is higher than in normal tissues. Chronic stimulation of tissues by the process of hypoxia could explain cancer development. But let's say that the benign growth is in its early stages, and the immune system starts to fight off the abnormal but non-cancerous areas. The following can then happen: Cells in the central areas begin to die off, and due to inflammation of the surrounding areas of the growth, a scar reaction is created, walling off the growth, leading to the development of a cyst (a walled-off fluid filled space) or nodule (a solid mass or lump).

For whatever reason, if this "walling-off" function of your immune system does not work properly, the growth continues to expand, moving into surrounding areas, or spreads to distant parts of the body. This is when cancer begins.

In men it's a given that as you age, the prostate enlarges, or some men will go on to develop prostate cancer. But notice that the incidence of OSA and heart disease goes up at this age as well. Traditionally, older men are thought to go to the bathroom more often as a result of prostate enlargement, but recent studies have shown that many of these men also had OSA. Countless studies also report improvement in nighttime arousals and the need to urinate after treatment for sleep-breathing disorders. The same applies to children and bedwetting as well. An interesting article revealed that almost 80% of nighttime arousals due to the urge to urinate in men and women are actually due to sleep disorders, particularly OSA.[7] Are heart disease, OSA and prostate enlargement separate, independent processes, or could they be related by one common link?

This concept of cancer or benign enlargement from a sleep-breathing perspective has significant implications. Obviously, we can't screen every person in this country for sleep-related breathing problems, but we could screen certain cancer patients (breast, colon or prostate) for sleep-related breathing problems and treat them simultaneously along with the regular treatment options. There's stronger reason to screen men with enlarged prostates for OSA. This could in theory improve quality of life measures as well survival rates in cancer patients.

As I mentioned earlier, having a cancer diagnosis in itself is very stressful. Even if you are not too stressed, your family and friends are going to be anxious about you, feeding into your own low-grade stress state. So improving sleep quality alone may not work all the time. But again this brings up the age-old question: Does stress aggravate or cause cancer? Ultimately, it doesn't matter, since one just feeds the other. Regardless of which came first, you should address both issues simultaneously.

We often hear of someone with terminal cancer who was miraculously cured, either with or without any medical intervention. It's well-known in traditional as well as complementary and alternative medical models that emotions and the mind play a very important role in cancer. From a sleep-breathing-cancer standpoint, I'm willing to bet that the people who had these "miraculous" cures, by addressing their anxiety and stress issues via whatever means (meditation, yoga, prayer, etc.), influenced their immune system to successfully fight the cancer.

Another issue that is important is that if you do have cancer and you have a sleep-breathing problem (whether or not one caused the other), then in a hospital setting (especially after surgery) or in bed at home, you may be more often forced to sleep on your back, thus causing the raft of problems outlined previously in this book. It is possible that this simple act could actually lead to the progression of your cancer or to other complications during your hospital stay.

In summary, I'm not proposing a radically new way of treating cancer. I'm definitely not saying that a sleep-breathing condition causes cancer. However, if you are predisposed genetically, and start out with a few cancer cells that normally would have been eradicated by your immune system, having an underlying sleep-breathing condition could allow the benign or cancerous cells to survive. What I am suggesting is that it may be beneficial to look outside of our traditional models of disease. The sleep-breathing paradigm allows us to view cancer in a totally different way. Hopefully, this "concept" can be applied to real-life people with beneficial results.

16 Sleep & Breathing: The Connections of the Heart

Kyle is a 55 year old man who came to see me after many months of chronic throat clearing, hoarseness and a lump sensation in his throat. His exam revealed laryngopharyngeal reflux disease, with irritation of his voice box with acid from the stomach. He tells me that he suffered from a heart attack at age 45 and is on medications for high blood pressure and high cholesterol. He snores like a chainsaw, just like his father did before dying from a heart attack at age 56.

To be honest, I really didn't want to write this chapter. In fact, I dreaded writing about the thousands of studies that link sleep-related breathing disorders and heart disease, high blood pressure, heart attack and stroke. But since the above conditions are the most important and potentially most deadly complication of OSA, I feel an obligation to at least summarize what's out there in sleep apnea research.

One of my major frustrations is that despite the overwhelming evidence that having OSA can cause, if not trigger, high blood pressure, heart disease, heart attack, and stroke, 80–90% of people with OSA in this country remain undiagnosed. As I stated previously, most physicians still never consider the possibility of OSA in someone who does not fit the classic profile of the three Os: Older, Overweight, and Obnoxious snorer. If you add Male and Snoring, you'll get the acronym MOOOS. Despite repeated studies that show even young thin women who don't snore can have significant OSA, physicians would rather focus on the end results, such as high blood pressure, depression, diabetes, etc.

Whenever I see an older man with heart disease, high blood pressure, high cholesterol and diabetes on fifteen different prescription medications, it brings tears to my eyes. If his doctors had only asked about his heavy snoring and fatigue twenty years ago, or considered that his father snored heavily and died of a heart attack in his late forties. I know skeptics will say that he would have developed all these things anyway and that there's no way to prove that treating him for OSA would have prevented the progression of all these medical conditions. My answer is that knowing what we know now, it's inexcusable for someone like this not to undergo a sleep study to rule out OSA. Even if treating the apneas doesn't totally cure all the presenting conditions, it can dramatically improve the quality of life, and perhaps cut down much of the daily medication consumed. Medications can come with numerous side effects that only add to the total physical and psychological load on the patient.

Let's begin by describing a typical middle-aged, mildly over-weight male who snores. The latter is so bad that his wife has to use earplugs. She also elbows him so that he turns over onto his side, which lessens his snoring. He feels exhausted at the end of the day, which he attributes to many hours at a stressful job. His father snored heavily and also had high blood pressure and heart disease, before dying of a heart attack in his early sixties. He sees his primary care physician for an annual check-up, and is found to have slightly high cholesterol levels (the bad kind) and his blood pressure is creeping up as well. Fortunately, his doctor listens to the man's off-handed remark about his wife being bothered by his snoring, which triggers the possibility of OSA, which he heard about at a lecture the previous day on heart disease. He orders a formal overnight sleep study, which reveals that his patient stops breathing 55 times every hour for an average of 22 seconds. The longest one lasted for 41 seconds. His blood oxygen saturation levels, which should normally be in the mid to upper 90s, dipped to as low as 81%. He is offered CPAP treatment and does very well, waking up much more refreshed in the morning, and with much more energy later in the day. He begins to exercise more and is able to lose some weight, and eventually brings down his cholesterol levels, and his blood pressure as well. I will discuss CPAP treatment in a subsequent chapter.

Obviously, this is an ideal scenario, but it's a good example to analyze. Ceasing to breathe multiple times throughout the night as described above leads to a number of different physiologic consequences. Periods of low oxygen levels (along with elevated carbon dioxide levels) triggers a stress response by activating blood gas level sensors in the body, which constricts blood vessels. During an apneic episode, tremendous vacuum pressures are created (up to −80 cm of water pressure), which prevents proper blood flow to the heart, which ultimately results in less blood being pumped out of the heart. After the apnea ends, chest pressure returns to normal, and a sudden increase in blood flow through the heart along with constricted blood vessels can lead to a severe rise in blood pressure. Also, when the brain senses that you are not breathing (due to high carbon dioxide levels), it wakes you up from deep sleep to either light sleep or complete arousal, which also can raise your blood pressure. If this continues over months or years, the elevated blood pressure can carry over into the daytime. Also, these rapid pressure fluctuations can cause injury to the lining of the blood vessels, which can promote or aggravate heart disease or stroke.

Low oxygen levels can also encourage white blood cells to attach to the lining of blood vessels, releasing damaging free oxygen radicals. Hypoxia is also associated with an increase in many inflammatory markers, such as tumor necrosis factor α, interleukin-6, and C-reactive protein (CRP), possibly all due to white blood cell attachment to damaged blood vessel lining. CRP has been found to be elevated in people with OSA. Treating these patients (for OSA) lowered the CRP levels back to normal. Interestingly, CRP is also one of the most useful markers for cardiovascular disease and risk. There are some studies suggesting that there is an increased risk of clotting in people with OSA.

Leptin, which is a hormone produced by fat cells that suppresses appetite, is elevated in both overweight people and people with OSA. This implies that the brain is resistant to the action of this hormone, which leads to continued hunger despite eating a large meal. High levels of leptin also have been shown to promote platelet clotting, which increases the risk of heart attack or stroke. And as I described in a previous chapter on sleep and weight, if you gain a few pounds, it can narrow your throat, leading to even more apneas.

OSA can also prevent glucose from being optimally absorbed into cells by making your body less responsive to insulin. As a result, glucose stays in your bloodstream, which has many detrimental effects, such as the development of diabetes.

Your cholesterol levels can also be affected by OSA. It's been shown that OSA is associated with a lower than normal HDL cholesterol (the good kind), which can be raised significantly with appropriate OSA treatment.

The combination of a stress response, blood vessel lining injury, inflammation and leptin/glucose/insulin imbalance can lead to a number of clinical problems. The strongest evidence we have for cause and effect is that OSA can cause high blood pressure. There are some authors who are bold enough to state (hypothetically) that untreated OSA may be a major cause of all high blood pressure problems. I've put these studies to use in my practice: Whenever I see a young adult with unexplained high blood pressure on medications, I always ask about sleep-breathing issues. Sure enough, the vast majority are found to have OSA on a formal sleep study. Even if they don't have it initially, many years later, after they've gained some weight, a repeat study shows that they have OSA. Not surprisingly, recent weight gain is a common event in someone with newly diagnosed OSA.

OSA can also aggravate, if not cause, heart rhythm problems, heart failure, heart disease, heart attack and stroke. Imagine if your heart is struggling to pump blood during the apnea episodes, and attempting to cope with the effects of adrenalin associated with the accompanying stress response, which stimulates the heart muscles. Think about what that would do to your heart. Since the heart is controlled by electrical currents, any degree of extra stimulation could potentially aggravate or cause rhythm problems, whether it goes too fast, or too slowly. Even if you don't have significant OSA, multiple arousals and stressful stimulation associated with UARS could aggravate rapid heartbeat or anxiety issues.

If you have OSA, you have about a 40% higher chance of having a heart attack, compared with someone that doesn't have OSA. Your chance of having a stroke is about 50% higher. OSA has been shown to be an independent risk factor for stroke.[1] Snoring alone is linked to an increased risk of stroke.

Despite all the above evidence, leading medical researchers continue to say that we need more definitive studies before OSA is recognized at the same level as high blood pressure or diabetes. Hopefully, you as the reader will take this information and encourage your doctors to take it more seriously.

17 Hormones: The Lowdown on Sleep

Emily is a 49 year old woman on thyroid medication for hypothyroidism. She gained significant weight after a prolonged course of oral steroids for asthma about two years ago. Ever since gaining weight, she's feeling more tired, and recently, her doctor told her that her blood sugars were a little high. She's constantly hungry, especially at night and frequently craves fatty and sweet snacks before bedtime.

THE BODY HAS MANY WAYS of communicating between distant organs or tissues. One way is to send signals through your nervous system, which includes sensory, motor, or involuntary nerve fibers. Another way of signaling is to send chemical messengers called hormones through the blood stream to distant parts of the body. For example, your master hormone gland (your brain) sends thyroid stimulating hormone (or TSH) through the bloodstream to your thyroid gland to make thyroid hormone. The thyroid hormone that's produced feeds back to the brain, which raises or lowers TSH, keeping thyroid hormone production at an appropriate level. Thyroid hormone is what ultimately controls your body's metabolism.

Many of my patients who come to see me for routine ear, nose or throat problems also happen to have various hormonal issues such as hypothyroidism, diabetes or menopause. Not unexpectedly, the patient attributes his or her main problem to the one hormonal deficiency, such as hypothyroidism or low insulin. But knowing what we know about all the hormones in the body, it's safe to say that every hormone in your body is completely interdependent. Supplementing your low thyroid levels with thyroid hormone doesn't really treat what's causing the low thyroid levels to begin with. This "unknown cause" is most likely causing other obvious or subtle hormonal imbalances as well.

Looking at this issue from a sleep-breathing perspective, it's not surprising that many of these patients also have hormonal imbalances. A stressful physiologic state that results from multiple arousals or frequent obstructions can definitely cause not only a nervous system reaction, but also a hormonal change as well.

So what happens when you experience poor sleep for a period of months or even years? No matter how many hours of sleep you get each night, quality is compromised if your upper airway anatomy is prone to obstruction during deep sleep.

Let's ignore for a moment all the other reasons for poor sleep, such as staying up late, feeding the baby, etc. Let's assume that you are able to go to sleep at a reasonable time and are able to get eight hours of sleep, but continue to wake up tired and groggy. Initially, the effects of these multiple arousals may only affect you at night while you are sleeping, but eventually, you'll feel it during the day.

If the body registers that it's under stress during sleep, the brain will respond in two ways. First, it activates the sympathetic (fight-or-flight) part of the nervous system, which tenses the blood vessels, speeds up the heart and breathing rate, along with other associated effects. It also releases a substance called corticotropin-releasing hormone, or CRH, from the brain. CRH travels to the pituitary gland, which stimulates adrenocorticotropic hormone (ACTH) production, which subsequently travels via the bloodstream to the adrenal glands (located above the kidneys), and glucocorticoids (mainly cortisol) are released as a result into the bloodstream. Cortisol helps to mobilize energy reserves, mainly glucose, into the bloodstream. It also stimulates appetite. CRH helps to activate your fight-or-flight response, which promotes adrenaline release from your adrenals glands as well, in addition to stimulating the heart and constricting blood vessels.

The hormonal and nervous system's response to stress leads to a number of other effects. Leptin is a hormone produced by fat cells that tells the brain that the stomach is full. This hormone therefore plays an important role in appetite control. Sleep deprivation and stress can lower leptin levels, which increases appetite. Leptin levels rise at night during sleep, and a direct correlation exists between the number of hours slept and the level of leptin in the body. The more you eat during the day, the higher your leptin levels will rise at night. Cortisol, released as a result of the stress response, not only makes you hungrier, but also makes your brain less sensitive to leptin.

In experimental rats, sleep deprivation increases both appetite and stress levels which, in turn, lowers leptin levels. Sleep deprivation also raises hypocretin levels, which has a stimulatory effect on the brain, as well as increasing appetite. Coincidentally, most narcoleptics are found to have a deficiency of hypocretin in their brains. Narcoleptics suffer from unexpected, brief episodes of deep sleep during the day. A low level of hypocretin may explain why narcoleptics suffer these anomalous sleeping episodes.

Interestingly, leptin and cortisol play reciprocal roles in the body. When one is high, the other is low. Sleep disruption was found in one human study to lower leptin levels in the evening, with a corresponding rise in cortisol levels. This can have the effect of stimulating appetite in the latter part of the day.

Sleep restriction is also found to lower thyrotropin-releasing hormone (TRH) levels from the hypothalamus. TRH normally travels to the pituitary gland, which releases TSH. In this same study, the normal peak in TSH that is characteristically seen in the late evening was found to be blunted. This may explain why some people with sleep-breathing disorders have hypothyroidism.

Sleep deprivation also lowers the body's ability to absorb glucose—this is called glucose intolerance. Insulin is needed to help the body absorb glucose into the cells. As a result of glucose intolerance, insulin is increased in response to the elevated levels of glucose in the bloodstream. In both sleep deprived people and insomniacs, evening cortisol levels were found to be elevated, in addition to lowered glucose tolerance. Cortisol makes fat cells less sensitive to insulin. Insulin and cortisol synergistically can lower leptin, which can lead to an increase in appetite.

Ghrelin is another hormone that is produced in the stomach and which stimulates appetite. It has the opposite effect of leptin; ghrelin increases just before eating and drops after a meal. Not surprisingly, sleep deprivation raises ghrelin levels, increasing appetite.

But there's more: Stress is found to suppress luteinizing hormone (LH) and follicle stimulating hormone (FSH) in both men and women. These hormones are vital for proper reproductive health and functioning. Interestingly, endorphins (the so-called "happy" hormones responsible for a runner's high), can also suppress luteinizing hormone releasing hormone (LHRH) which, in turn, lowers LH.

In men, the parasympathetic nervous system (the relaxation part) is responsible for arousals and erections. The sympathetic (stress response) handles orgasm and ejaculation. I'll leave it up to you to decide what may happen if there is too much stress in a man's life.

Similarly, bladder function is also controlled by these two complementary nervous systems and can malfunction as a result of stress. Lastly, cortisol blocks the action of vasopressin (antidiuretic hormone, or ADH) on the kidneys to reabsorb water. As a result, urination increases.

But at this point you may be thinking that, yes, stress and sleep loss can make me more hungry, but the last time I got stressed, I had no appetite. This can be explained by the fact that when you undergo an intensely stressful event, CRH is released within seconds whereas glucocorticiods can take minutes to hours to respond. The initial burst of adrenaline from CRH release decreases once the stress event is over, but the glucocorticoid response can take hours to dissipate.

The initial CRH release tends to suppress appetite, whereas gluco-corticoids stimulate appetite. As the initial stressful event subsides, glucocorticoids predominate and glucose levels can remain elevated for minutes to hours.

This concept implies that one long period of intense stress (run-ning away from a tiger) is better for your overall state of health than multiple intermittent short stresses (multiple stressful events all day at work), since a lingering glucocorticoid release can not only make you more hungry, it also causes you to prefer starchy or sugary foods. This is why in the immediate period just after a stressful episode, we take comfort in comfort foods.

The hormonal mechanisms described here are only the tip of the iceberg. My main point in writing this somewhat complicated but thankfully brief chapter is to illustrate that sleep, breathing, weight, and appetite are all marvelously interrelated. People with wide jaws and open breathing passageways will be relatively less susceptible to the sleep-breathing dilemma of modern society. Changing one element can change everything else. Until modern times, there was a harmonious balance between each of the four elements, but now with the added stresses of modern society, along with presumed narrowing of our anatomic breathing passageways, it's no wonder that we can suffer from the full compliment of these ailments.

18 Stressed Out, Tired & Sleepy?

Robert is a 44 year old man who complains of chronic sinus pressure and pain, along with chronic severe fatigue and intermittent joint pains and muscle aches. He recently underwent a full examination with blood work, which were all unremarkable. His doctor raised the possibility of CFS, and wants him to get formally evaluated for this condition. He complains that he is a poor sleeper, never feels refreshed in the morning, and is exhausted by the mid-afternoon. He notes that he suffered from "mono" in his early 20s, from which it took him about six months to fully recover. He drinks three cups of coffee in the morning.

IT SEEMS LIKE EVERYONE is tired these days. Physically, mentally, emotionally and psychologically tired. We all have our excuses, including a stressful job, working long hours, or money issues. But it seems like this problem is much worse now than it was fifty years ago. Maybe it's the price we pay for modernization or improved information technologies. Some may argue that the world has not changed, but that we're not able to adapt or adjust quickly enough. Why are we so overworked, overstressed and overweight?

We take it for granted that in this day and age, we're all going to feel tired to some degree no matter how we live our lives, but there are some people who are so tired, that it literally consumes them to the point where they can't function normally. If you are one of these people, you know that you never feel refreshed in the morning, no matter how many hours of sleep you may have had. Many of you toss and turn at night, waking up frequently, or are not able to fall asleep at all. Could it be that major presentation in the morning, your new mattress, or the taxes you have to pay? Or is it your bed-partner's snoring, or your cat that's keeping you from sleeping fully at night?

When you wake up in the morning, despite the lingering fogginess and fatigue, you drink your Starbucks 20 ounce coffee and rush to work. You're constantly on the move, interacting with people, making calls at a hectic pace, going nonstop all day long. After eating a quick lunch, you make it through the afternoon, but only by drinking a few more cups of coffee and munching on donuts that your boss brought. When you get home, you're too exhausted to go to the gym. You have dinner around 9 P.M. and go to bed at 10 P.M. You toss and turn. When the alarm goes off at 6 A.M., you're barely able to get out of bed.

To compensate, many people go to the gym every day. For some, they find it almost an addictive process. When this occurs, they often feel lousy and lethargic even if they miss out on just one session. Others end up taking a nap for an hour or so as soon as they get home from work, and by the time they wake up, it's 10 P.M. After a quick dinner, they try to go to sleep, but aren't tired. So they stay up until 2 A.M. but have to wake up at 6 A.M. to go to work. Needless to say, they are exhausted. After work, the cycle starts all over again. Usually they're able to catch up with their sleep on the weekends, but now even that is not as easy as it used to be.

If you find yourself caught in this never-ending cycle, you may find that you're more moody or irritable, snapping at the smallest things. You're more forgetful and can't concentrate as well as you used to. Various medical ailments may appear, such as recurrent headaches, sinusitis, indigestion, diarrhea, or general aches and pains. You may start waking up to go to the bathroom more often. You may also begin to have anxiety issues during the day, where your heart races and you sweat profusely for no apparent reason. Alternatively, you may feel depressed and avoid doing things you once enjoyed.

At this point, you may decide to go see your doctor about your problem, because you know something is wrong. Usually, the exam and all the tests will come back normal. You're told there is no obvious illness that could account for your problems. Frustrated and exhausted, you look up all your symptoms on the internet and you are bombarded with scary-sounding names that make you even more stressed.

Believe it or not, many of my patients have gone through very similar experiences. Usually, they'll come in for their recurrent sinus infections or chronic throat pain. Many will have already been given one of many diagnoses such as chronic fatigue syndrome (CFS), fibromyalgia, irritable bowel syndrome (IBS), hypothyroidism, or TMJ disease. The more doctors you have consulted for your seemingly endless array of problems, the more likely you'll end up with one of the above conditions, depending on what your main symptoms are. If you have chronic diarrhea, and your gastrointestinal evaluation is normal, you'll be given a diagnosis of IBS. If you have chronic pain in many parts of your body, you'll be classified with fibromyalgia. Often it becomes a simple process of choosing your most dominant symptom and labeling you with that disorder.

One surprising observation that I noticed many years ago regarding all the above types of patients is that with very few exceptions, almost every one of them was unable to sleep on their backs. The remaining few who could sleep on their backs did so due to a back, shoulder or neck pain or injury. For most patients, one or both of their parents were heavy snorers and displayed one of the complications of OSA, such as high blood pressure, depression or heart disease. Most of these patients were young and thin, and there was always some sort of triggering event that started the problem, such as a major cold or infection, a very stressful life event, an accident, or mild weight gain. Pregnancy or changing to a more sedentary job are two other common reasons for a change in sleep habits.

Whenever I examine the above patients' breathing passageways with my fiberoptic camera, I almost certainly find the airway to be narrowed, especially when they're lying flat on their backs. The opening between the base of the tongue and the back of the throat is often only one to two millimeters wide. This structural phenomenon creates the basis for the sleep-breathing paradigm that I have described repeatedly throughout this book. Whether you are aware that you are waking up or not during the night, you are still prevented from reaching, and maintaining, deep quality sleep.

If you have UARS and an arousal occurs during REM sleep (when your muscles are relaxed the most), you may wake up suddenly from either a nightmare or very vivid images. This makes sense since you will remember your dreams more clearly when awakened during REM sleep. Over the years some people have told me that they used to have very vivid and crazy dreams, but now that they are older (and heavier with OSA), they don't dream at all. This implies that their sleep-breathing problem is worsening, and they are not able to reach REM sleep at all. Many of my patients who are treated successfully for OSA report that they begin to dream again.

So what is the medical effect of all these arousals? As described in the previous chapter on breathing, multiple obstructions and immediate arousals can lead to a stress response, which stimulates your "fight-or-flight" response. Hormonally and neurologically, your body thinks it's under attack or ready to fight, releasing adrenaline. If obstruction occurs, and breathing ceases for ten to thirty seconds followed by waking out of sleep, two processes are put in place. One is the stress response described above. The second is a lowering of blood oxygen levels, known as hypoxia. As I mentioned in a previous chapter, hypoxia can lead to a variety of cardiovascular problems and possibly cancer-promoting processes.

It's not uncommon for many of these patients to already have been diagnosed with CFS, fibromyalgia, irritable bowel syndrome, or hypothyroidism. I'm not discounting the validity of any of these conditions, and I'm not saying that inefficient sleep is the *cause* of all these problems. I'm only suggesting that if you have any one of these conditions, having a sleep-breathing condition can definitely aggravate the underlying problem. But at a certain point, it doesn't matter which comes first—one aggravates the other. What I see quite often is that if the sleep-breathing problem is addressed thoroughly, the other conditions can improve significantly as well.

If you look at all the books out there on CFS, there are two types of treatment philosophies: the magic bullet and the shotgun approach. The magic bullet approach can be anything from a particular nutritional deficiency to adrenal gland "burnout." The shotgun approach is probably more realistic, as it admits that we just don't know exactly why CFS exists. Many medical conditions that could result in CFS have been described in various textbooks and other resources. With thorough and extensive detective work and numerous tests, the most likely sources are treated simultaneously.

One popular condition that explains chronic fatigue is the "adrenal burnout syndrome." It's stated to be a 21st century stress syndrome. Common symptoms include severe fatigue, trouble getting out of bed, lack of energy, decreased energy, decreased sex drive, decreased ability to handle stress, dizziness and lightheadedness when standing up, low body temperature, a propensity for colds and infections, depression, allergies and increased pre-menstrual syndrome (PMS) symptoms and menopausal dysfunctions. Does this sound familiar? It's not just a coincidence that these are the same list of symptoms in patients with upper airway resistance syndrome. I'm willing to bet that the vast majority of sufferers are not able to sleep on their backs, and they are poor sleepers, tossing and turning, with frequent nighttime arousals. Inquiries about the parents of such patients often leads to the discovery that one or both were chronic snorers, and one or more have one of the consequences of OSA, such as depression, high blood pressure, obesity, heart disease, heart attack or stroke.

Adrenal burnout syndrome is a condition where the adrenal glands are unable to produce sufficient amounts of cortisol and DHEA, another hormone made by the adrenal gland. I have seen some dramatic responses to administration of prednisone, which is a synthetic oral form of cortisol. Many of these patients also have hypothyroidism, or clinical symptoms of hypothyroidism without any abnormal thyroid blood tests. This can be explained by the fact that a stress response will suppress thyrotropin-releasing hormone or TRH (which normally stimulates thyroid stimulating hormone), and cortisol prevents proper conversion of T4 to T3 in the body's cells. With this syndrome, there is either insufficient thyroid hormone, or what is produced doesn't get converted to a form that the cells in the body can use effectively. This is critical since low thyroid hormone levels can lead to symptoms of fatigue and weight gain.

The sleep-breathing paradigm presented in this book is not meant to be an answer for all the ailments mentioned to date. For some people, having true hypothyroidism can aggravate weight gain, which can promote a sleep-breathing problem which can, in turn, promote weight gain. Despite taking thyroid medications, many are still tired and continue to gain weight. By taking measures to treat any existing sleep-breathing problem, you can lessen the fatigue and slow down the weight-promoting process. But for many others, it's clear that a sleep-breathing issue is the main source of the problem. In the OSA research literature, there's significant controversy over whether hypothyroidism causes OSA or OSA causes hypothyroidism. Obviously having an underactive thyroid can make you gain weight, and weight gain can aggravate OSA, but using the sleep-breathing paradigm, you can also argue that sleep-breathing problems can aggravate hypothyroidism.

Lastly, your body doesn't care where the stress is coming from. If you already have a sleep-breathing issue, then you'll have a low-grade stress-response cycle spinning inside your body at all times. You may compensate by drinking lots of coffee, or exercising and staying active. But any external source of stress whether emotional, physical or psychological can speed up this internal cycle, aggravating your condition even more. This can cause physical changes in your body, which can feed back to your mental and psychological state, which feeds the stress response further.

Another concept in stress physiology that should be mentioned is the concept of stress and the sequential timing of the multiple responses that follow. Robert Sapolsky in his book, *Why Zebras Don't Get Ulcers*, posits that under times of stress, your gastrointestinal system literally shuts down, with less protective mucous production in your stomach, or recruitment of immune cells to your small intestine. Once the stressful event is over, and you begin eating again, a large meal will activate the acid-secreting cells of the stomach. But with a reduced protective mucous barrier to keep the acid from burning a hole through your stomach, an ulcer can form. A rapid influx of blood and nutrients causes a rise in oxygen free radicals, a dangerous byproduct of oxygen metabolism. Normally, the body makes substances that eradicate these free radicals, but if your gut has been sleeping, it won't have a store of these protective agents when oxygen starts pouring in again. Another possible injury mechanism that Sapolsky describes is due to poor circulation resulting in microscopic strokes, leaving tiny areas of dead tissue in the gut, which can cause problems such as an ulcer or an infection.

Another important point that Sapolsky brings up is that it's not so much the stressful event and the body's response that causes the injury or illness, but that once the stress is over, it's the residual effects of the stress response and the body's process of repairing itself that causes the greatest amount of damage.

Take, for example, the stomach ulcer situation. It's not the stress, but the period afterwards that is the critical time for injury. In fact, studies have shown that in the initial period of intense stress, your immune system is actually stronger. This makes sense, since you'll need to run away or heal a cut. The same goes for a stressful event leading to a surge in cortisol and activation of the sympathetic nervous system. It's ultimately not the initial stress response that is potentially damaging, but the prolonged corticosteroid/cortisol response that over time with repeated episodes that causes injury and damage to your body.

So with repeated, chronic stress in our daily lives, along with advancements in modern conveniences and technology that keeps us awake at night, we are definitely not only sleeping less hours, but the hours that we sleep are becoming less efficient. If you factor in the sleep-breathing paradigm with its underlying anatomic principles as an aggravator of this process, things look very bleak. However, I will discuss how we can deal with these issues in later chapters.

19 Flashing Lights, Ringing Ears & Plugging Noses

Jason is a 69 year old man who complains of chronic ringing in both ears that seems to have been getting worse over the past two years. His hobby is ice sculpting and Jason admits that he sometimes forgets to use ear protection. A hearing test shows severe nerve deafness at 4 kHz in both ears, suggesting that it may be due to chronic noise exposure in the past. He has slept on his side all his life, but since his hip surgery about two years ago, he's been forced to sleep on his back, and has noted that he is more tired than usual in the morning.

INCLUDED IN THIS CHAPTER are various ear, nose and throat conditions that are best discussed collectively, as they apply to sleep-breathing disorders.

Tinnitus (Ringing in the Ear)

Tinnitus, or chronic ringing in the ear, is one of the most frustrating conditions that an otolaryngologist must deal with on a daily basis. Although there are millions of research dollars devoted to this topic, there hasn't been any significant advance in the past few decades. Either you are told you just have to live with it, or you undergo a million dollar work-up and then are told you have to live with it.

The classic type of ringing is a constant humming, ringing or hissing, in one or both ears, that is bothersome to the point where it keeps the person up at night. There's another kind, called pulsatile tinnitus, in which blood flow turbulence is audible to the sufferer. Classic tinnitus can range from nuisance value to a major ordeal, sometimes leading to the point of suicide. For most people it's something that comes and goes, noticed more often when they are under stress or have trouble sleeping.

The cause of tinnitus is still unclear. There are many theories that speculate on its origin. Some theories propose that the condition is due to inner ear nerve damage, where the sufferer hears phantom sounds. Others state that the brain misinterprets signals from the inner ear. These are overly simplistic explanations, with dozens, if not hundreds, of variations and modifications.

In more severe cases, depression often coexists. This is why in some patients, treatment with an antidepressant medication sometimes helps the tinnitus. But this again brings up the chicken and the egg question: Does tinnitus cause depression or does depression cause tinnitus? We may never know the full answer, but I think we can all agree that one can definitely aggravate the other.

So how does the sleep-breathing paradigm fit into this discussion on tinnitus? Remember I mentioned a study demonstrating that any form of sleep deprivation can lead to a lowering of the pain threshold? This means that someone who does not get enough sleep, or is not allowed to sleep effectively, will sense pain much sooner and at a more magnified level compared with someone who sleeps well. This concept can be extrapolated to all the other senses of the body.

Imagine if you had some form of subtle damage to your inner ear, and a mild, barely perceptible tone was audible as a result. In the beginning, it didn't bother you that much, but as you began to lose sleep, all your senses become more aware, and any little noise, light, movement or ringing will bother you and keep waking you up. This leads to more inefficient sleep, perpetuating this all-too-familiar vicious cycle. I recently had a patient who complained of constant ringing in her ears for the past two years. It didn't greatly annoy her, except occasionally when it was quiet, just before going to bed. I found out that she was a life-long stomach sleeper, but had to switch to her sides due to a back problem. When I asked her when she switched her sleep position, she thought about it for a few seconds, and with a sudden sense of clarity, admitted that it occurred about two years prior. Hence the advent of the tinnitus had coincided with the change in sleep position.

There are some obvious causes of ringing, such as chronic loud noise or music exposure, aspirin or similar medication use, certain toxic medications, but for many causes of tinnitus, there is no obvious answer. However, one thing that I see almost consistently is that people with tinnitus do not sleep well. They tend to toss and turn, and rarely are able to sleep on their backs. Does this sound familiar to you?

Sudden Hearing Loss (Nerve Deafness)

Fortunately, sudden one-sided nerve deafness is uncommon, but it does occur in rare cases. In many situations, the hearing loss does improve significantly, but in others, the person will have permanent one-sided hearing loss. Treatment with various medications (in particular prednisone, an oral steroid), has been shown to help restore hearing loss to a relatively normal level. There is now controversy over how well prednisone works or, in fact, whether it works at all. Regardless, there are three general theories as to why this occurs.

The first one is the infectious theory. There are many viruses that can infect the inner ear, including the common cold. The problem is that there's no way of proving that the inner ear is infected in these cases. Just sampling or culturing the inner ear could lead to a worsening of hearing loss. A second theory involves an autoimmune condition, where the body attacks itself, in this case, the target is the inner ear. Again there is no way of proving this directly, but clues may exist elsewhere in the body. Thirdly, there is the vascular insufficiency theory. Again for unknown reasons, the small arteries that lead to the inner ear are either blocked, or clot off. There is no way of proving this conclusively. Regardless of which reason is correct, the end result is inflammation. Inflammation causes more swelling. This is why prednisone helps sometimes because it assists in reducing swelling. It's important to note here that this type of hearing loss is different from a middle ear infection that produces another kind of hearing problem, called conductive hearing loss. Typically, in this scenario, there is fluid or pus in the middle ear that is responsible for diminished hearing.

Applying the sleep-breathing paradigm, where chronic low-grade stress exists, the involuntary nervous system will divert all blood flow and energy to the central muscles, the heart and the brain, effectively preventing the "end organs" and other "low-priority" organs and body parts from receiving normal blood flow. Not too surprisingly, the inner ears are considered an "end-organ." Cold hands and feet are another result of this blood shunting process. Instead of giving oral steroids, maybe stress reduction and relaxation techniques would better address this problem (see later chapter on conservative treatment options).

Hyperacusis (Noise Sensitivity)

Another variation on the tinnitus problem is a severe sensitivity to certain noises, pitches or voices. These particular sounds are very painful and uncomfortable, sometimes to the point of being debilitating. Imagine every little sound on the street in the city bothering you like finger nails on a chalkboard. If you apply the sleep-breathing paradigm to this situation, it makes sense. The nervous system is heightened and hypersensitized due to poor sleep, and if your hearing is abnormally good, certain sounds will be very uncomfortable due to the body's oversensitivity to noise. If you are prevented from getting deep sleep or under more stress than your usual baseline state, the noise sensitivity worsens as a result.

Photophobia (Light Sensitivity)

Photophobia, or sensitivity to light, is a common condition that is seen with a variety of conditions, such as migraine headaches or meningitis. Since so many people with UARS have migraine headaches, this condition deserves some comments. Again, using the sleep-breathing paradigm as the basis for a hypersensitive nervous system, if your eyes are particularly sensitive, then any excessive light will bother you. Think of a migraine attack as an episode of involuntary nervous system outburst, hypersensitizing or stimulating your eyes, your nose, your ears and your sinuses. You may also feel nausea or vomit. Your eyes can tear up. Stimulation of the sinuses and nose result in swelling. The latter causes nasal or sinus congestion, leading to symptoms that sound like routine sinusitis. Hyperacusis is also common during a migraine attack.

This condition can also be extrapolated to hangovers. Headache, photophobia and hyperacusis are common symptoms of a hangover. After even one drink, some people are more susceptible to hangovers. Again, if you have a propensity for tongue collapse, then alcohol is more likely to relax your throat muscles, aggravating obstruction and arousals or apneas, leading to significantly less efficient sleep. Less efficient sleep can lead to light and sound sensitivity. We know that morning headaches can also occur with OSA. Either by direct neurological stimulation of the sinuses or via direct acid exposure of the sinuses due to tongue collapse and arousals (or apneas), closure of the sinuses can definitely aggravate sinus headaches.

Nasal Packing

A variety of ear, nose and throat conditions require nasal packing, the most common reason being for severe nosebleeds. Traditionally, a long strip of gauze (about six or more feet) is placed inside the nose on one side or, if necessary, both. These days, a compressed dry sponge that expands once inside the nose is used. Nasal packing is also commonly undertaken after any type of nasal or sinus surgery.

If you've ever had nasal packing on both sides, it's a miserable experience. Not only are both nostrils completely closed for two to three days, but removal is unpleasant as well. Why is it so uncomfortable to begin with? As I alluded to previously, nasal congestion can aggravate OSA or arousals. Possessing a susceptible facial anatomic configuration will likely result in a temporary case of OSA while the nasal packs are in place. This is similar to suffering from a simple cold, with a blocked nose, causing you to toss and turn because you can't sleep.

I remember reading an old study that showed that college students who have their noses pinched closed are found to have significant OSA when they undergo a formal sleep study. More recently, patients who had nasal packs for severe nosebleeds were found to have significant OSA.[1] This is why I stopped using all forms of nasal packing, even after routine nasal and sinus surgery, with rare exceptions. Besides causing a vacuum effect downstream and aggravating tongue collapse, there are also many reflexes that link your nasal breathing and reflexes to your lungs and heart. One traditional warning about posterior nasal packs, which are placed in the back of the nose to control severe bleeding, is that there have been reports of heart rhythm problems, heart attacks, or even death associated with their use. This was blamed on the naso-cardiac reflex. Stimulation of nerve endings in the back of the nose is thought to cause heart rhythm irregularities. That is why people with posterior nasal packs are recommended to be placed in the intensive care unit to monitor breathing and heart rate.

An alternative explanation for the occurrence of difficulties with nasal packing is that total nasal obstruction aggravates further tongue collapse, leading to apneas, causing an excitability of a heart deprived of oxygen, thus producing the potential of a heart attack. In addition, if the person normally prefers to sleep on their side or stomach and suddenly is forced to sleep on their back, apneas and obstructions are likely to occur, stressing the heart. You can imagine that it's very difficult to sleep on your back or side when lying in a hospital bed, with all the wires and monitors attached to every limb, and with the head of your bed tilted up somewhat. I'm not saying that the naso-cardiac reflex does not exist; in fact, during residency, I remember one patient who was intubated (had a breathing tube in his windpipe so OSA was not an issue) suffered from a heart attack just after his posterior nasal packing was removed.

Chronic Sinusitis

I alluded previously to the causes of chronic nasal irritation from acid regurgitation and swelling of the nasal and sinus mucous membranes as a result of recurrent tongue and palate obstruction and arousals. Needless to say, chronic nasal irritation and swelling can not only cause nasal congestion, but also sinus infections. This can happen occasionally, on a frequent basis, or never go away after just one infection. In patients with chronic sinusitis (with documented objective evidence on a CT scan and non-response to long courses of oral antibiotics), treatment with an acid reducer (omeprozole 20 mg twice daily for 3 months), produced significant, but modest symptom improvements.[2] Of note, treating doctors did not look for OSA in these patients. Another study showed that treating OSA patients with omeprozole (20 mg twice daily for 4 weeks) significantly lowered the apnea index by 25% and three out of ten patients were considered "treatment responders."[3] This was one of the major papers that sparked the idea for my sleep-breathing paradigm.

Another observation from my own experience over the years was that, of the total number of patients who undergo functional endoscopic sinus surgery or septoplasty, between 5 to 10% return complaining of recurrent or persistent symptoms (such as nasal congestion or sinus pressure and pain). Many of these patients improved with medical treatment. Of the remaining patients who still did not get better, almost 80% were found to have significant OSA, as determined by a formal overnight sleep study.[4] This is a surprisingly high number, since only about 4 to 25% of the population are estimated to have OSA. As a result of this finding, I don't have to perform as many sinus surgery or nasal procedures anymore, because by treating the underlying OSA, these symptoms usually improve without further intervention.

20 Your Stuffy Nose

Margaret is 35 and remembers having a stuffy nose for many years. When she was younger, a doctor told her she had a deviated septum. She underwent rhinoplasty 10 years ago to make her nose look better. She tried using multiple allergy medications including antihistamines and nasal allergy sprays, but they only helped temporarily. She went to see an allergist and after testing, was told that she did not have any significant allergies.

THIS CHAPTER ADDRESSES THE VARIOUS conditions that can cause nasal congestion, since proper breathing through your nose is critical to what occurs lower down in your throat. Many people with sleep-breathing problems have some degree of nasal congestion, and in general, this issue should be dealt with first before addressing other areas of the throat, such as the palate or the tongue. The reason for this is that any degree of nasal congestion can create a vacuum effect downstream, causing the tenuous palate or tongue structures to collapse more easily. This is similar to sucking through a flimsy straw with the tip pinched closed, causing the middle part of the straw to collapse.

As you are aware, noses come in varying shapes, sizes, and configurations. It also doesn't matter how big your nose is—it's the width of your internal breathing passageways that determine how well you'll breathe. Unfortunately, opening up the nose via medical therapy or even surgery has been found to "cure" OSA in only 10% of people. Patients will definitely feel and breathe better, but it's uncommon that their sleep apnea is addressed definitively. However, I have seen many of the people in the "10%" group with dramatic significant improvement. Besides breathing better for the first time in years, opening up the nose can allow the person to tolerate and benefit from other treatment options for OSA.

Deviated Nasal Septum

One of the more common reasons for a stuffy nose is due to a deviated nasal septum. A "septum" is a term that describes a structure that acts as a wall or separator between two cavities. Your heart has one too. No one has a perfectly flat or straight septum. All septums, by definition, have slight irregularities or curvatures.

There's a lot of confusion about what the septum is. As you can see from Figure 20.1, it's quadrangular in shape, where the front cartilaginous part juts out to the tip of the nose, and meets the nasal bones in the midline higher up. The upper-rear and lower-rear portions are made of thin bone. Near the back of the nose, the septum ends. Along the side-walls of the nasal cavity are three (sometimes more) structures called turbinates. These structures are wing-shaped and normally help to smooth, warm, and moisturize the air you breathe. It also produces a thin mucous blanket that traps dust and other particles. Eventually, this mucous blanket gets slowly pushed to the back of your nose and is eventually swallowed. The average person produces and swallows about three cups of mucous every day.

It used to be thought that a deviated septum occurred due to some form of trauma, occurring during birth or due to physical injury later

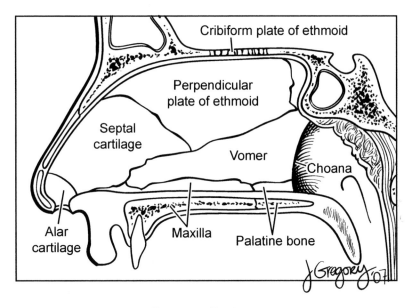

Figure 20.1 Nasal septum

in life. We now know that people who were born via c-section with no history of nasal trauma can have a deviated septum. It is also possible to have a curved shape, have bony or cartilaginous spurs, or the septum can even be displaced off the floor of the upper jaw where it normally sits.

Surgery to fix a "deviated septum" is usually considered after medical options like avoidance measures, allergy medications, or even allergy shots have failed. The procedure is relatively minor, takes about 30–60 minutes, and you can go home a few hours after the surgery.

Many surgeons traditionally place a tampon-like plug inside the nose after nasal or sinus surgery to prevent bleeding. Ever since I stopped using nasal packing of any kind for this procedure many years ago, patients are much happier since they are able to breathe immediately after the operation. My reasoning for not using packing is that in many of my patients, having a completely blocked nose can aggravate or worsen any underlying OSA. If you've ever had your nose packed for any reason (nasal surgery, nosebleeds, etc.), it's a miserable experience. I still remember the time I broke my nose at age six and having my nose packed for a few days after corrective surgery. Taking out the packing was definitely an unpleasant memory.

Flimsy Nostrils

In some people, the space between the nasal septum and the soft part of both nostrils is either too narrow to begin with, or they collapse partially or completely during inspiration. In many cases, this can be seen years after reduction rhinoplasty, where the nose was made smaller or narrowed for cosmetic reasons. Now that we know that this can occur, a good rhinoplasty surgeon should be able to prevent this from happening. Occasionally, people can possess a naturally thin and floppy nostril structure.

Another common reason for flimsy nostrils is due to a narrow upper jaw. The width of your nose follows the width of your jaw. If the angle between the midline septum and the nostril sidewall is more narrow than normal, then it's more likely to collapse with any degree of internal nasal congestion. It's not surprising that people with sleep-breathing disorders will typically have narrower jaws, and thus more susceptible to nostril collapse. Certain ethnicities are also more prone to this phenomenon than others.

There are two cartilages that make up the soft part of the nostril: the lower lateral and upper lateral cartilage (Figure 20.2). During rhinoplasty surgery, a portion of the lower lateral cartilage is frequently removed for the purpose of narrowing the lower third of the nose. The results may look great initially, but over time, the nostrils become pinched in and collapse during inspiration, causing nasal congestion.

One way that you can easily tell if you have this problem is to perform the Cottle maneuver: Place both index fingers on your face just beside your nostrils. While pressing firmly against your face and simultaneously pulling the skin next to the nostril apart towards the outer corners of your eyes, breathe in quickly. Then let go and

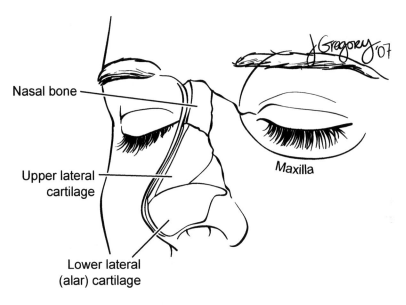

Nasal bone

Upper lateral
cartilage

Maxilla

Lower lateral
(alar) cartilage

Figure 20.2 Nasal anatomy

breathe in again. If there is a major improvement in your quality of breathing while performing this maneuver, then you have what's called nasal valve collapse.

The simplest way of correcting nasal valve collapse is by using nasal dilator strips, or Breathe-Rite® strips. If you do the Cottle maneuver and there is no significant difference in your breathing, don't waste money buying these strips. If you perceive an improvement in your breathing, you can continue using the strips at night while you sleep. For some people, these "strips" are not strong enough to hold up the nostrils, or may cause irritation to the skin. Athletes sometimes use this product to enhance nasal breathing.

There are also many other "internal" options available over the counter, including metal springs or plastic cones that are placed inside the nostrils. People tolerate these particular devices differently, so the only way to know if you'll like them is to try them. Three examples are Breathe With EEZ™, Nozovent®, and Sinus Cones™.

Note that almost everyone has some mild degree of nasal valve collapse—if you sniff in hard enough, your nostrils will collapse. Even during quiet breathing, due to the pliability of the nostrils, there is a mild degree of narrowing. However, if you have a cold or allergies, this causes congestion inside the nose, which creates a vacuum effect, allowing your nasal valves to collapse even more. You may have also noticed that when you are exercising or angry, your nostrils can widen. This is due to the nasal dilator muscles that can be useful in certain situations.

To find out if your nasal valve collapse is from weak or flimsy cartilages or is aggravated by internal nasal congestion, you can spray nasal saline (which is a mild decongestant) into your nose. If your nostrils doesn't collapse as much, then you need to address your internal nasal congestion first. A stronger over-the-counter medication that you can use is oxymetazoline, which is a topical spray decongestant. There are many brand name and generic versions that are sold that contain this ingredient. It's very important that you don't use this medication for more than two to three days—otherwise, you may get addicted to it.

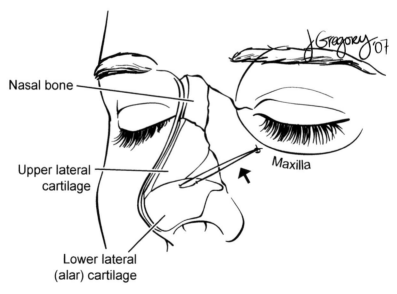

Figure 20.3 Nasal valve suspension suture (arrow)

If you want a permanent solution to this problem without having to use dilator strips or internal devices, the only option is surgery. The traditional way of dealing with this issue is to perform a kind of reconstructive rhinoplasty surgery, usually by taking small portions of your nasal septal cartilage or ear cartilage and placing in underneath the weakened portions of your nostril walls. A newer, simpler way of addressing this problem is by attaching a permanent suture just underneath the eye socket and tunneling the suture under the skin and looping it around the weakened area to suspend the nostril to prevent collapse (see figure 20.3).[1]

Wings in Your Nose

Another common source of nasal congestion is from swelling of your nasal turbinates, which are the wing-like structures on the side-walls of the nasal cavity opposite the septum. Turbinates are comprised of bone on the inside and mucous membrane on the outside (Figure 20.4). The area just underneath the mucous membrane is filled with blood vessels which can swell significantly, similar to the way the penis can enlarge. As the turbinates swell, the air passageways narrow further, especially if you have a mildly deviated nasal septum, and particularly if you have nasal valve collapse. If you are sensitive to pollens, dust, mold, weather changes or animals, then the turbinates inside your nose will swell slightly, producing excess clear mucous. Colds, infections, weather changes and even acid from the stomach or migraines can aggravate these structures, causing blood to fill up and clog up your nose. If you have allergies, by taking avoidance measures and treating the allergies appropriately, this problem is usually correctable.

If conservative treatment including prescription allergy medications don't work, various surgical options are available from very conservative 5 minute in-office procedures to more aggressive procedures that are performed in the operating room. These procedures are usually performed alongside a septoplasty to improve nasal breathing.

What's the Nasal Cycle?

Your nasal turbinates swell and shrink alternating from one side to another every few hours. This is controlled by the involuntary nervous system automatically, and it's so subtle that you won't notice it in general. However, if you have a cold or allergies, and both turbinates are slightly swollen, you'll notice that your nose gets blocked from side to side, one nostril at a time. Also, if you lay down, due to blood pooling in the turbinates and due to gravity, you'll get even more congested.

Nasal Polyps

I want to briefly mention the word "polyp" as used in regard to the nose. A polyp is a generic medical term meaning a swelling or growth that protrudes from a mucous membrane. Polyps in the colon are usually benign, but cancers can arise from them as well. In the nose, however, they are usually benign, and are rarely cancerous. Typically, polyps in the nose arise from chronic irritation, inflammation or infection. One of the more common causes is allergies. Chronic allergic inflammation of the nasal mucous membranes can lead to low grade swelling in certain areas of the nose, particularly near the sinus passageways. Continued swelling can lead to blockage of the nasal passageways, the sinus passageways, or both. Other causes of swelling, such as a simple cold, can lead to similar processes.

One of the most common misunderstandings that I see by both doctors and patients alike is that they think that swollen turbinates are polyps. The nasal turbinates can swell so much that you can sometimes see the reddish-pink, fleshy grape-like mass through your nostrils. Once decongested, they shrink dramatically and the air passageways open up again.

If your nose is stuffed up in any way, air can't reach the roof of the nose, where small smell-sensing nerves sprout down from the brain through tiny holes in the plate of bone that separates the roof of the nose from the undersurface of the front of the brain. When this happens, you lose your sense of smell. And if you can't smell, you can't taste as well either.

Sinusitis

If you suffer from sinusitis, this can cause nasal congestion and inflammation combined with post-nasal drip, sinus pressure, and pain. Put simply, pure misery. Sinus infections typically follow either a routine cold or allergy attack; they cause both swelling and blockage of the sinus passageways, leading to negative pressure initially and, if allowed to progress, can turn into a full-blown sinus infection, with yellow-green discharge, fever and severe facial pain. Your teeth can also hurt since the roots of the upper molars jut up into the floor of the maxillary sinuses. Similarly, dental pain can sometimes feel like sinus pain.

Fortunately, most cases of sinus congestion will eventually go away. The body has a remarkable ability to take care of these issues without any intervention. Sometimes bacterial infections occur, and with proper conservative treatment using saline and decongestants, the infection gradually resolves. Rarely, you may need an antibiotic to control stubborn bacterial infections.

What's in the Back of Your Nose?

The back of the nose is called the nasopharynx, and this is where your adenoids sit (see Figure 20.4). The adenoids are similar to tonsils, but comprise a single gland located in the upper-back section of the nasopharynx. In most cases, the adenoids slowly shrink away. Some younger adults can have persistently enlarged adenoids, which can lead to nasal congestion when inflamed.

Off to the side of the nasopharynx, there are two little slits that connect via thin tubes to the middle ear cavities. These are the Eustachian tubes. Whenever you swallow or chew or yawn, attached muscles tug on the Eustachian tube opening to equalize pressure

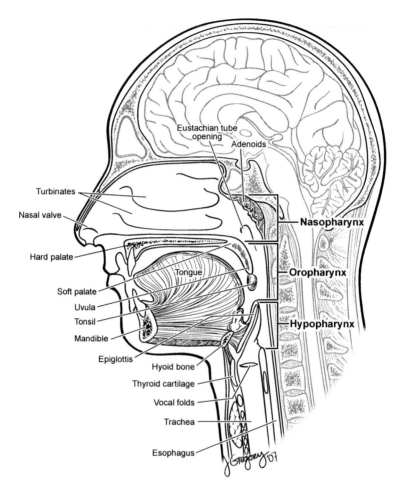

Figure 20.4 Nasal sidewall

between the nose and the middle ear. In some people this pressure equalizing mechanism doesn't work properly and they tend to have chronic ear problems.

Below the nasopharynx is the soft palate, which separates the throat from the nasal passages while swallowing. Muscles in the soft palate also tense to open the Eustachian tubes during swallowing, as well as to maintain food and water in your throat and propel it down into the esophagus and thus to the stomach.

As you can see from the above discussion, there are a number of various reasons for having a stuffy nose. But the most common reason for nasal congestion that I see routinely is due to inefficient breathing and poor sleep. Yes, structural reasons, allergies, or nasal polyps can definitely block your nose, and these issues must be dealt with appropriately. But in general, it's the inflammation that's created by a combination of your hypersensitive nasal nervous system and possible stomach acid regurgitation into the nose from multiple obstructions and arousals, that causes nasal congestion. Without addressing this underlying source of inflammation, correcting a deviated nasal septum or treating for nasal allergies will only provide a temporary solution.

21 | Your Annoying Snoring Problem

Elizabeth is a 49 year old woman who complains of severe left ear pain since getting an ear plug stuck in her ear two days ago. She normally uses ear plugs to help muffle her husband's intense snoring sounds at night. She's a light sleeper, and is more tired in recent months, possibly due to a new, more stressful job. After removing the soft ear plug from her ear in the office, she felt much better.

IF YOU ARE THE VICTIM OF A SNORING BED-PARTNER, you are not alone. In a study by the National Sleep Foundation, 67% of adults reported that their partner snores.[1] Many couples sleep separately in an attempt to minimize the problems caused by chronic loud snoring. It's estimated that about 20% of men and 5% of women in their thirties snore, but these figures rise to 60% of men and 40% of women in their sixties.[2] About 35% of habitual snorers are estimated to have OSA, which is a staggering percentage of the population.[3] However, of most concern is the fact that about 80–90% of people with OSA are not diagnosed, implying that a significant number of snorers have undiagnosed OSA.[4] This is important because untreated OSA is known to be linked to an increased risk of developing high blood pressure, depression, obesity, heart disease, heart attack or stroke.

Whether or not you snore, you should read on. As I mentioned in the breathing chapter, you don't have to snore to have significant sleep-breathing problems, including OSA. If you suffer from chronic fatigue, lack of energy or many of the other problems mentioned in previous chapters, then this may be an important chapter for you later in life. Or you could be sleeping with someone who snores. By reading this chapter, you could potentially save his or her life.

Snoring is no laughing matter. Although some doctors claim that there can be such a thing as "benign snoring," I think that all snoring implies partially obstructed breathing. Imagine the last time you had a cold and your nose was partially blocked. You could still breathe, but you were uncomfortable. This also explains why people tend to snore more when their noses are stuffy. The fact that you are snoring means that somewhere between your nose and voice box, there is a narrowed area of soft tissue that has constricted to the point where air squeaks through and the palate vibrates. This is not normal. This process can cause various degrees of deep sleep interruption, leading to poor quality sleep for you as well as for your bed-partner.

If you snore, that means that you're still breathing. But consider this: If you stop snoring, then the situation can be more dire—you can be obstructed and not breathing at all.

From Snoring to Obstruction

Let's say that you go to sleep on your back. Remember that during deep and especially REM sleep, your throat muscles relax, predisposing you to either partial or total obstruction. When your throat muscles are partially relaxed, and as your tongue begins to fall back, air is drawn through your throat at a faster rate (like sucking through a flimsy straw), creating a vacuum effect, narrowing the soft palate structures. When the area behind the palate narrows to a certain point, the soft tissues begin to flutter, and you begin to snore. If your bed-partner is bothered, then he or she will elbow you, and you will roll over onto your side, lessening the loudness of snoring (bruised rib syndrome). If you remain on your back, snoring will increase in intensity as you progress through your sleep stages from light to deep sleep. At a certain point, especially in deep sleep, your throat muscles relax completely and you will stop breathing.

Once this occurs, two things can happen: After you try to take a few breaths inward, your brain senses that you are not breathing or are about to stop breathing and wakes you up subconsciously to light sleep or a semi-awake state. If you stop breathing for greater than ten seconds and then wake up, you just had an apnea.

Why Snoring Matters

Snoring is accompanied by a variety of health problems, from mild to severe. Evidence suggests that the vibrations caused by snoring damages the nerve endings in the soft palate, weakening muscle tone, thus further aggravating snoring.[5] This is like your hands going numb after using a sander or handheld massager. Studies also report that loud sound vibrations could cause carotid artery wall trauma and rupture of plaques in rabbits, which has implications for humans.[6] This is one way that we suffer from strokes.

In addition to the consequences of forceful sound vibrations, the loudness of the snoring sounds can cause additional problems. The loudest recorded snore was measured at 103 decibels, which is louder than standing next to a diesel bus engine. Regulations require that ear protection must be worn for industrial jobs once the sound level reaches 90 decibels. Interestingly, the wife of one of the world's loudest snorers was deaf in one ear. No prizes for guessing in which ear she was deaf.

Because snoring is a predictor of multiple health problems, one way of roughly predicting your own future health is to look at your parents. If your father snores like a train, has depression, high blood pressure, and had a heart attack at age 51, then your snoring may mean that you are at risk for similar problems in the future.

There are hundreds of studies that link snoring and a higher incidence of high blood pressure, heart disease and stroke in adults,[7-9] as well as behavioral problems, learning difficulties, and asthma in children.[10,11] If you have a large population of snorers, a significant fraction of these people will also have OSA. This means that it's not so much the snoring that's causing all the problems, but that the presence of OSA within the snoring group will skew the numbers, causing an association between snoring and all the above medical conditions.

It's important to also bear in mind that OSA is not something that you either have or don't have. As you can see from Figure 21.1, everyone is on a continuum. Simple snorers are at the left of the line, but as you either gain weight or age, you can move up the line to the right, towards clinical OSA.

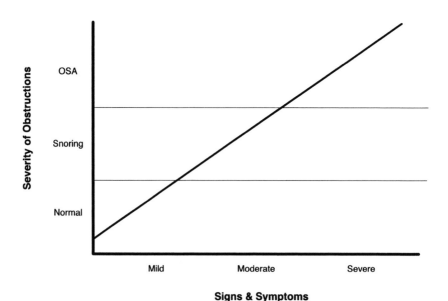

Figure 21.1 Sleep-breathing continuum

Not So Simple Tips for Snorers

If you look at various medical websites on the internet or in brochures, you will see the same list of bulleted points listed below to help with your snoring. They include:

- Eat healthily and exercise
- Lose weight
- Avoid tranquilizers, sedatives, antihistamines, or older-style sleeping pills before bedtime
- Avoid alcohol or a heavy meal for at least three to four hours before bedtime
- Practice regular sleep patterns
- Sleep on your side or stomach

These tips may seem like common sense ideas, especially the ones about eating the right foods, exercising, and maintaining a healthy weight. Also, alcohol or any medication which relaxes your muscles can make you go to sleep faster, but they worsen the quality of your sleep.

There are over 300 patents registered to treat snoring. If you read the product packaging or their website testimonials, it may seem that their product is the "cure" for snoring. The problem is that it only works for some people. And even if it does work to help the snoring, you may be delaying getting proper diagnosis and treatment for OSA.

Some common devices that are marketed for snoring include nasal dilator strips, a throat lubricant spray, and a pillow. A recent study objectively showed that these three devices did not significantly improve snoring.[12] I have some patients that do find them useful, but the improvement is not consistent enough for me to recommend. However, there are some instances where after a thorough medical examination, I may recommend a nasal dilator strip, especially if you have nasal valve collapse, as described in Chapter 20.

Another common recommendation for snorers is to sew a sock with a tennis ball to the back of your pajamas while sleeping. In theory, this sounds great, but in practice, all it does is to prevent you from sleeping on your back and ultimately delays the diagnosis of sleep-breathing problems. There are even devices that detect when you are snoring and wakes you up. Yes, it stops the snoring, but you're still waking up. In essence, your bed-partner's elbow can do the same thing for essentially no cost.

In my experience, people try many of the over the counter options and even some of the conservative measures, with limited success. Many just give up and accept the fact that snoring is just a routine part of life and just deal with it. I mentioned in a previous chapter that one of the trends in new housing construction was a request for two separate master bedrooms.[13] The major reason for this request was due to bed-partner snoring. Obviously, snoring by itself will not break up a relationship, but if there are other issues that are not addressed, sleep deprivation due to a snoring partner can aggravate any pre-existing problems. For a more detailed discussion on how to treat snoring, please refer to Appendix A.

By whatever means snoring is initiated, it is a sign of health problems down the road. The next time you hear someone snoring, whether it's your loved one or your next door neighbor, before covering up your ears or banging the walls, have that person talk to a doctor first. You could be saving his or her life.

Section 3

Modern Day Solutions For Your Sleep-Breathing Problem

22 How Do I Know If I Have a Sleep-Breathing Problem?

I F SOME OR MANY OF THE SYMPTOMS described in this book sound familiar, you may be wondering by now if you have a sleep-breathing condition. I don't want to use the words *disorder* or *disease*, since by the sleep-breathing paradigm's definition, all humans are susceptible to this condition to various degrees. Having temporary obstructions and arousals can be a mere inconvenience, but if this condition continues or progresses over a significant time period, you will feel it one way or another. If you are on the far right of the sleep-breathing continuum line (Figure 22.1), then you may have OSA, which is a well-defined clinical condition that needs attention. However, many of you will be to the left or middle of the line, with varying degrees of severity or number of symptoms. The following questions in this chapter will help you determine where along the continuum you lie.

Do you prefer to sleep on your side or stomach?

As I've mentioned before, if you have a sleep-breathing condition, you are more likely to sleep on your side or stomach. The one exception is when you have a good reason where you must sleep on your back due to a physical injury or pain (shoulder or neck injury, back pain, etc.), when in the past you loved to sleep on your side or stomach.

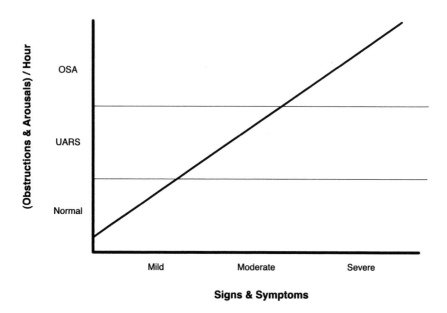

Figure 22.1: The sleep-breathing continuum

What's the quality of your sleep?

Do you wake up refreshed, ready to go in the morning, or do you have a hard time waking up, despite sleeping between seven to nine hours? Do you need a cup of coffee to get going in the morning with additional cups later throughout the day? Are you exhausted later in the afternoon or in the evening, or do you have to take naps in the afternoon? The answers to these questions will provide clues on how well you sleep in terms of sleep efficiency. Obviously, if you are only sleeping four to five hours a night, increasing your sleep time gradually and improving your sleep hygiene first may have a positive effect on your day. If, however, after changing your sleep pattern and these questions still elicit a "yes," then you may have a genuine sleep-breathing problem.

Is your nose stuffy or runny all the time?

Is your nose more stuffy at night when you go to bed? Have you tried over-the-counter or prescription medications with limited success? Have you undergone any nasal surgery in the past? Sleep-breathing problems can frequently aggravate nasal congestion, and vice versa.

How often do you wake up at night?

Do you ever wake up choking or gasping for air, or in a state of panic? What sleep position are you in when you wake up? People with sleep-breathing problems tend to wake up many times throughout the night, either consciously or subconsciously.

Do you dream regularly?

Do you dream at all? Do you ever wake up and remember wild or vivid dreams? Depending on where you are in the sleep-breathing continuum, you are more likely to have vivid dreams if you are towards the left side of the sleep-breathing diagram, and unlikely to dream at all if you are to the right of the line. You'll remember your dream more vividly if you wake up in the middle of a dream.

How often do you have to go to the bathroom?

If you drink lots of water, then you may have to wake up often to go to the bathroom. But consider that a sleep-breathing condition can also promote more urine production.

Do you ever wake up sweaty or have hot flashes during the day?

As I alluded to in the menopause chapter, men can have these same symptoms as well, especially when they are sliding up the sleep-breathing continuum to the right.

Do you have trouble falling asleep, or have trouble getting back to sleep once you wake up in the middle of the night?

How often have you taken sleeping pills for this situation? Stress and other factors can aggravate insomnia, but a sleep-breathing problem can make it worse.

Does drinking alcohol at night make you feel more groggy and tired in the morning?

For those of you who have experienced a hangover, the obvious answer is yes. But since alcohol also relaxes the muscles, including those in the throat, your sleep quality may worsen dramatically due to more frequent obstructions and arousals. Most people with this condition know not to drink at night.

Do you have to exercise every day?

If you exercise regularly, do you *have* to go every day, or can you miss a few days once in a while? If you miss one or two days, do you feel miserable and foggy-headed? Many people with sleep-breathing issues have to stay active, or they begin to feel drowsy and are unable to focus or concentrate.

Do you have cold hands or feet?

Some people can have warm, numb or sweaty hands or feet. All these symptoms result from a disordered nervous and vascular system in your extremities. If you are older and don't have cold hands, did you have the condition when you were much younger? As you move to the right of the sleep-breathing continuum, cold hands when younger generally go away as you get older, especially if you gain weight.

Do you have low blood pressure?

Even if your blood pressure is normal, do you get lightheaded or dizzy easily when you stand up suddenly? If you now have high blood pressure, did you have low blood pressure when you were much younger? Similar to the cold hands situation, low blood pressure generally improves to normal as you gain weight, and can even lead to high blood pressure later in life.

Are you slowly gaining weight?

Have you recently gained weight that you can't take off, no matter how much you exercise or diet? Did the weight gain occur after a major life event, such as pregnancy, an accident, or surgery? Many patients report sudden or progressive weight gain after these events, or even after a bad cold or flu which led to periods of inactivity. Any of these events can trigger or aggravate an underlying sleep-breathing condition, with worsening sleep quality, leading to less physical activity and hormonal factors that promote weight gain.

Do either of your biological parents snore?

If so, do they have a history of any the following: high blood pressure, diabetes, obesity, heart disease, heart attack or stroke? Do you have a sibling with any of the above features? What about your aunts and uncles, or your grandparents? Having a father that snores like a chainsaw doesn't automatically mean that you'll end up the same way, but there is a possibility, since you share the same genes.

Just How Sleepy Are You?

Questionnaires can be useful aids in determining the presence of a suspected sleep-breathing disorder. A common questionnaire that is given by many sleep physicians is the Epworth Sleepiness Scale. It's a very quick eight part tool that's used to screen for any possible sleep-breathing problems. There's some controversy over its usefulness, but I find it helpful as a screening tool, if used in light of the big picture (see Figure 22.2). If your score is 10 or above, statistically, you have a high likelihood of having a sleep-related breathing condition, especially OSA. The problem with this questionnaire is that it's more accurate when the score is very high, but not that helpful if the score is low. There are many other reasons to have a high score due to reasons other than OSA, such as insufficient sleep or narcolepsy.

In other words, if your score is 22 out of 24, I'd be surprised if you don't have some sort of a sleep problem, but if your score is 4, you could still have a sleep problem.

Epworth Sleepiness Scale

How likely are you to doze off or fall asleep in the following situations, in contrast to just feeling tired? This questionnaire refers to your chance of falling asleep, according to your usual way of life, for about the last week or two. Even if you have not done some of these things recently, try to estimate how they would have affected you during the last two weeks.

Use the following scale to choose the most appropriate number for each situation.

Scale:
0 = No chance of dozing
1 = Slight chance of dozing
2 = Moderate chance of dozing
3 = High chance of dozing

Situation:

Situation	Chance of dozing
Sitting and reading	0 1 2 3
Watching TV	0 1 2 3
Sitting inactive in a public place	0 1 2 3
As a passenger in a car for one hour without a break	0 1 2 3
Lying down to rest in the afternoon when circumstances permit	0 1 2 3
Sitting and talking to someone	0 1 2 3
Sitting quietly after lunch without alcohol	0 1 2 3
In a car, while stopped in traffic for a few minutes	0 1 2 3

Total Score _____

Scoring:
7 or less: You have a normal amount of sleepiness
8 to 9:   You have an average amount of sleepiness
10 to 15:   You may be excessively sleepy depending on the situation and you may want to seek medical attention.
16 and up: You are excessively sleepy and should seek medical attention.

Figure 22.2 Epworth Sleepiness Scale

There are dozens of other, more complicated questionnaires that are used in clinical research, but the above example is a simple way to alert both the patient and the physician to the possibility of a sleep-breathing problem.

Examining Your Airway: What to Expect

The next step in determining whether or not you have a sleep-breathing problem is to look inside your throat. Although the general examination can be performed by any physician, the endoscopic examination is best performed by an ENT physician.

The following is an overview of such an exam if you were a typical patient in my practice. I begin with an examination of your tongue position in relation to the free edge of your soft palate. This determines if the snoring comes solely from the palate or the palate and tongue together. It also has implications for surgery (described in Chapter 25). I then place a thin camera through your nose and examine the area of your voice box that I see behind the back of the tongue. I perform the Mueller's maneuver by pinching the nose closed and asking you to sniff in strongly through the nose (Figure 22.3). In people with lax or redundant soft palate tissues, I will see a circumferential collapse, either partially or fully.

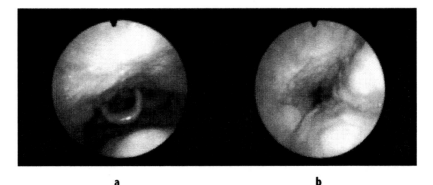

a   b

Figure 22.3: Mueller's maneuver before (a) and after (b)

I also will ask you to try to snore. If you are able to snore, I will usually see the soft palate fluttering with the snoring efforts. The soft palate is the most common area that produces the classic snoring sound. However, other areas of your throat, such as your tonsils, tongue and epiglottis (the upper part of your voice-box) can vibrate as well.

Next, I concentrate on the opening behind your tongue and down to your voice-box. From above, I note the relative position of your tongue in relation to the area on top of your voice-box. I may be able to see anything from the entire v-shaped vocal folds to almost nothing. Passing the camera further into the oral cavity, I examine the vocal folds and voice-box in detail. I look for nodules or polyps, and in particular, I look for swelling and irritation in the back part of your voice-box, which is seen in people with throat acid reflux (LPRD).

The next part involves having you lie flat on your back in the exam chair (see Figure 22.4a). This time, I notice again where your tongue is in relation to your voice-box. In some people who have narrow dental arches while in a seated position, there exists a noticeable collapsing of the tongue due to gravity when lying down. In other cases, the tongue may have initially been pushed well back in the mouth to begin with, so when lying flat on the back, there is nowhere for the tongue to go except to occlude the airway passage.

The last part of the examination involves thrusting the lower jaw forward (Figure 22.4b). This causes the jaw to pull on the genioglossus muscle, which is attached to the back of the tongue. This opens up the space behind the tongue significantly in some people. Countless others have various gradations of the above. If you have a dramatic response to this maneuver, then one option for treatment is a mandibular advancement device. This is discussed in more detail in Chapter 24.

Depending on what your principal complaint is, and the overall picture that I have of your history and exam findings, I will make a recommendation as to whether or not a formal overnight sleep study is needed.

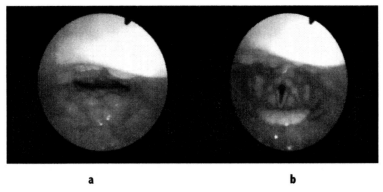

a   b

Figure 22.4 Airway opening lying flat on back (a), and with jaw thrust (b)

Testing for a Sleep-Breathing Problem

The standard overnight sleep study, or polysomnogram, involves monitoring a number of different variables, such as heart rate, oxygen levels, brain waves, eye, chin, leg, chest and abdominal movements. This is a comprehensive test that not only measures how well you breathe at night while asleep, but also measures your heart rhythms, leg movements, and sleep position. After a few days, enormous amounts of data are tabulated and analyzed, and sent to the referring physician.

Many people are hesitant or reluctant about going to a sleep lab and being told to sleep in a strange bed with many wires attached. Others are adamant that they will never fall asleep in that kind of environment. Despite all the apprehension, it's rare for anyone to go through an entire night without any useful data recorded. For a brief video of me undergoing an actual sleep study, visit www.sleep interrupted.com/video.html.

You may have heard about home-based sleep studies, which in theory should be more comfortable for obvious reasons. Many variations exist, from formal comprehensive studies (with multiple parameters, or channels), to a single channel (oxygen level or breathing only). Despite their obvious convenience, they are not as reliable or as accurate as a professionally conducted study at a sleep unit. Another major reason for not doing a home-based sleep study is that if one of the channel leads fall off, there's no technician to come in right away to replace the lead. If this happened at home with an important single lead, the entire study would be wasted. For this reason, when possible, I prefer to order an in-lab study. However, with technological advances, home-based studies should be more acceptable in the future.

Once I receive the sleep study report, I look over all the various results, but I initially focus on the apnea hypopnea index or AHI. An apnea is when you stop breathing completely for ten seconds or more and a hypopnea is a partially restricted breathing episode of more than ten seconds. I look at the AHI in the following situations: overall, REM, non-REM, supine (back position), and non-supine.

There are two kinds of apneas: obstructive and central. Most apneas due to anatomic narrowing are obstructive. Central apneas occur when the brain does not send a signal to the diaphragm and lungs to breathe, and is more commonly seen in heart failure.

If apneas are present on your sleep report, I then look at how long the apneas lasted, and how low the oxygen levels dropped. For people with severe OSA, there can be anywhere from 40 to over 100 breathing pauses per hour on average, each lasting 10 to over 30 seconds. If you do the calculation, someone with moderate OSA with an AHI of 30 and an average length of 20 seconds each means that you are not breathing for 20 minutes every hour! I have many patients whose numbers are well over 100 times per hour. These patients are not breathing for 30–40 minutes every hour. Anyone with significant OSA requires treatment, for reasons stated throughout this book.

At the other extreme, there are people who don't have any apneas or hypopneas, but have multiple obstructions and arousals, which don't qualify officially as an apnea. If you stop breathing 30 times every hour, but each episode lasts no longer than 9 seconds, then officially, your AHI score is 0. Most labs will tell you that you don't have OSA. The more advanced labs will calculate these arousals from non-apneic obstructions and add that figure to the total number of apneas and hypopneas, giving you what's called the respiratory disturbance index, or RDI.

This is where it gets frustrating. There's no set standard across different sleep labs defining how an RDI is calculated. Some centers use AHI and RDI interchangeably, and others report two different numbers.

Yet, after putting together all the information described in this chapter, you and I will have a discussion, either in person or on the phone, about the different options available.

In general, there's no one solution for everyone. Each patient has a unique anatomy from the nose to the throat. Everyone has different needs and expectations. I spend a great deal of time determining what improvements, if any, the patient wants from treatment. Some people don't want to be treated at all despite having severe OSA. The next few chapters detail all the different treatment options, from very conservative to more aggressive.

23 Taking Immediate Steps To Feel Better

IF YOU THINK YOU MAY HAVE a sleep-breathing condition, whether it's a mild problem or an emergency, the short answer to how you can begin to feel better is: it depends. It depends on where you lie along the sleep-breathing continuum.

The first part of this chapter describes conservative and simple commonsense ways of addressing sleep problems. I will then go on to discuss basic sleep hygiene practices that the vast majority of Americans typically don't, but should follow.

Go Get a Physical

If you haven't undergone a routine physical in a long time, get one. There are many other common medical problems (including anemia, hypothyroidism, etc.) that can cause you to feel tired all the time. But if everything comes back normal, then take a look at how you can improve your sleep. Many of you will be able to dramatically improve sleep quality with just simple changes. For others, you'll have to work a little harder, but believe me, it will be worth it.

One thing to note is that all these conservative options do help in varying degrees. These measures can only modify or lessen the physiological effects of frequent upper airway obstruction which only occurs at night. Some people will feel dramatically better, whereas others will feel only mild improvement. Some will feel nothing at all. The best way to know is to pick the options that are most appropriate for your situation.

Determine Your Optimal Sleep Position

As mentioned in Chapter 22, the first thing you should determine after your physical exam is to determine your favorite sleep position. If you used to sleep on your stomach, what prompted you to turn onto your back again? Did your grandmother tell you that it was healthy to sleep on your back, or did your dermatologist tell you not to sleep on your stomach to prevent wrinkles? Most of you are already sleeping on your side or stomach to compensate already so there's nothing more you can do. Your problems are occurring because you are obstructing and waking up despite sleeping on your side or stomach. Again, there's usually something that may have triggered the onset of symptoms despite continuing to sleep on your side or stomach. It may have been weight gain, a major infection, or the development of allergies.

If you are sleeping on your back, and are able to, try sleeping on your sides or stomach, whichever is more preferable. Experiment for a week at a time in different positions. See which position is most satisfying when you wake up in the morning. One old home remedy for snoring is to sew a tennis ball into a pocket on the back of your pajamas (or safety-pin a sock filled with a tennis ball). This in theory should prevent you from turning onto your back, not only helping with snoring, but for tongue obstruction and arousals as well. I even had one patient who is doing well using a backpack stuffed with tennis balls to keep himself from rolling onto his back. It doesn't work for everyone, but you won't know until you try it. Some people naturally prop themselves on pillows to sleep upright. If you do have a shoulder or neck injury, get that taken care of so that you can get off your back when you sleep.

Change Your Meal Times

If you eat late at night, adjust your schedule so that you don't go to bed for at least three hours after eating dinner. This is one of the most common habits that, if changed, can make a dramatic difference not only to the quality of your sleep, but how well you digest food. If you have food in your stomach when you go to sleep, acid and stomach contents can leak upwards more easily, even if you don't habitually obstruct. This is why propping yourself up with pillows works to some degree in gastroesophageal reflux disease (GERD), as opposed to laryngopharyngeal reflux disease (LPRD). In LPRD, one proposed explanation is that the upper esophageal sphincter is leaky, compared with a loosening of the lower esophageal sphincter in GERD. Regardless of sphincter function, a vacuum effect in the throat from tongue obstruction can overwhelm both functioning sphincters.

As described in previous chapters, any degree of acid (or pepsin or bile) can be very irritating to the throat. Stomach juices have even been shown to reach the lungs, sinuses and ears. This is why for some of you, modifying your diet can also make a big difference. Cut down on anything that includes caffeine, alcohol, chocolate, mints, spicy foods, and citrus products. I didn't say cut *out*, only to cut *down*. Use common sense. Instead of eating something spicy, choose something less spicy. If you already eat a very bland diet, then that's one less thing you need to worry about.

Many people with chronic hoarseness or throat irritation from LPRD suck on throat lozenges or candy that contains either menthol or mint. Your throat may feel better temporarily while you have the candy in your mouth, but it can aggravate your stomach later on.

Control Your Allergies

If you know that you have nasal allergies, or suspect that you do, then take measures to avoid things that aggravate the condition. Allergies can cause nasal congestion, which can promote throat or tongue collapse downstream.

First of all, find out exactly what you are allergic to. Some people know exactly what sets off their allergic reactions, such as cats, ragweed in the fall, or dust. For others, it may take trial and error. If you really want to know, then see an allergist for formal testing. I would not spend any significant amount of money on allergy prevention products without knowing that what you are buying is preventing what you are allergic to. For example, don't get dust-proof bed sheets or buy a HEPA air purifier until you are certain that you are allergic to dust. It sounds like common sense, but many people buy products that are useless for what's really causing their allergies.

As a last resort, you can try over-the-counter or prescription allergy medications. For simple allergies that cause nasal congestion, you'll need a medication that acts as a decongestant. An antihistamine alone will not work. Common generic over-the-counter ingredients include pills (pseudoephedrine, phenylephrine) or sprays (phenylephrine, oxymetazoline). There are also a number of homeopathic sprays or pills for allergies that may be useful. Different people respond differently to various medications. My philosophy about alternative or complementary medications is, if it works, keep using it. For a free brochure on how to choose the right over-the-counter medications, visit www.sleepinterrupted.com/otcmeds.html.

Nasal saline can also be useful to some degree since salt water acts as a mild decongestant. By opening up your nose and sinuses, you will feel better and breathe better, especially if you have any chronic nasal or sinus issues. This is why your nose is more open and hence clearer when you go swimming in the ocean. The downside of saline is that it needs to be used frequently, sometimes every 4–6 hours. There are a number of different ways of getting saline into your nose, from simple small plastic bottles to aerosol cans to a "Neti Pot," which is an ancient Indian nasal saline douching method. They all apply salt water to your nose, but via different means.

A more aggressive way of getting saline more forcefully into your nose is to use a Water-Pik machine fitted with a nasal adaptor (www. hydromed.com). You can make up your own saline solution, instead of buying packets. One simple solution is to add ¼ to ½ teaspoon of salt (sea salt, pickling salt or Kosher salt) with a pinch of baking soda in 8 ounces of warm water.

One thing I've noticed is how many people who have severe cat allergies continue to own cats. I've not come across one cat lover who was willing to part with their cat to get rid of their allergies. In this situation, a few options include keeping the cat out of the bedroom, using a desensitizing spray, and washing the cat monthly with distilled water, which removes the dried saliva residue that most people are allergic to. You can also get a good HEPA filter, especially in your bedroom. Lastly, allergy shots are an option.

Follow Your Circadian Rhythm

Now let's talk about some simple ways of improving your sleep without medications. To understand how we can do this, we first need to appreciate how our ancestors slept. Before they had electric lights or Blackberrys, people slept when it was dark and woke up when it was light again. They spent much of their time outdoors hunting, farming, or undertaking other forms of outdoor activities. They worked hard and played hard all day long, and once the fire in the chimney or pit went out, they all went to sleep at the same time.

Today, things are very different. Not only do we have light bulbs, but we also have the internet, telephone, television, and taxes to distract us and keep us up at night. Not only that, many of us skip breakfast and go to work in an office building, without any sun exposure, eat a quick lunch, and get home late, eating a big unhealthy dinner before going to bed. Some of us exercise just before going to bed. But going to bed is not necessarily the time that you fall asleep. If only we could sleep like a baby for the time that we are lying in bed. The problem is that along with the anatomic factors that prevent us from getting deep restorative sleep, our work habits, daily stresses, and other dietary and lifestyle factors contribute to further degrade our sleep quality.

Your sleep is controlled by an internal circadian rhythm. There are a long list of neurologic and hormonal messengers in the brain that act as a "clock" to tell the rest of your body when it's time to sleep and when to wake up. A consequence of these messengers is that body temperature also rises and falls in relation to your awake-sleep state. As your temperature rises early in the morning, you have an urge to wake up. It continues to go up throughout the day, and begins to fall late in the evening, which goes along with feeling sleepy. These internal wake-sleep mechanisms take cues from the environment and your habits: the amount and timing of sunlight exposure, what and when you eat, when you exercise, etc. Most people are most awake and active during the early evening hours.

Here Comes the Sun

Sunlight exposure is critical in promoting a state of wakefulness, especially in the morning and during the day. When your brain senses light shining in your eyes, it stimulates the wake response, and lowers melatonin, which is a major hormone produced in the pineal gland of the brain that makes you drowsy. Once there is no more light entering the eyes, melatonin levels begin to rise, making you feel sleepy. In this age of electric lights and indoor work environments, you can see why our sleep patterns are so dysfunctional.

Morning sunlight is about twenty times stronger than office lighting. Mid-day sunlight can be up to 200 times greater. Make an effort to get out of the office, especially during lunch time. Walk or cycle to work if you can. Make up any excuse to spend more time outdoors. If you wear sunglasses, try not to use them as frequently as they block light from entering your eyes; you may want to use a hat instead to shield the sun. If you absolutely can't get any sunlight, another alternative is to use a bright light box, especially in the early morning hours, and in the office as well. These are commercially available from $200–300. You'll need the 10,000 Lux (55 watts) full-spectrum bulbs. There are many different ways to use it for different purposes, but the simplest way is to use it while reading or eating early in the morning for 15 to 30 minutes. These lamps have also been used successfully to treat the winter "blues" for decades. They are also great for use when you have severe jet-lag.

Get Moving

Exercise is a great way to strengthen the "awakening" forces in many ways, one of which is by raising body temperature and delaying the drop later in the day. It's been shown that regular exercise increases time spent in deep sleep. It's best to exercise early in the morning (outside), but if you must exercise in the evening, make sure it's no less than two hours before bedtime. If you exercise just before bedtime, you'll delay the body's temperature drop, preventing you from falling asleep when you want to. For helpful tips on how you can begin an exercise regimen that's right for you, visit www.sleepinterrupted.com/getmoving.html.

One of the most common situations in my practice that I see is when someone comes home at 8 P.M. after work, exercises for an hour, eats dinner at 9:30 P.M., and goes to bed soon thereafter. If this sounds like you, no wonder you have a hard time waking up in the morning, and need a large cup of coffee before you feel awake. If you have a sleep-breathing condition, the situation is compounded even further.

Timing is Critical

Your sleep cycle is like a roller coaster. The higher (awake) you go, the faster and deeper you can go (sleep). If you wake up only half-way, you can sleep only half-way, so to speak. This is why many people who have outdoor professions tend to be able to sleep much more deeply. They are exposed to sunlight all day long, and if involved with manual labor, achieve much higher levels of wakefulness, which is then countered by a strong desire towards sleep later in the evening. This may be an over-generalization, but office workers tend to have more issues with insomnia and poor quality sleep than outdoor workers.

Personally, I've never been a morning person. I've always been a night-owl. Some of my best work is accomplished from 9 P.M. to 1 A.M. As I write this sentence, it's 11:04 P.M. I still vividly remember the best month of sleep I ever had, just before entering college. I took part in a cycling/camping trip from Richmond, VA to Boston, MA. We cycled anywhere from 50 to 100 miles every day. Despite the fact that we slept in tents most nights, I still remember waking up consistently around 7 A.M. without needing an alarm clock, refreshed, rejuvenated, and ready to go. The combination of exercise and sun exposure all day definitely strengthened the peaks and troughs of my sleep cycle.

Also, think about how much better you slept the last time you went on vacation. You may think that it's because you didn't have any stress and you could sleep in, but notice what you did while on vacation—you spent time in the sun, either on the beach or walking around in a new city, usually outdoors. These activities stimulate your wake forces during the day, which also strengthens your sleep forces at night. For some of you, however, if you have a sleep-breathing condition, you may never feel rested and refreshed, even if you sleep for ten hours.

Another bad habit is the concept of "catching up" on sleep on the weekends. By sleeping in another 1–3 hours, you're not following your body's internal sleep clock. It's as if you are flying across a few time zones every weekend. This also disrupts your sleep time in the evenings, delaying your sleep time on Sunday night, but you still have to wake up early on Monday morning. You go to work still groggy, and stay that way, until you "catch up" the following weekend. Make an effort to wake up at the same time every morning. If you can, exercise outdoors in the morning on the weekends.

A better way of "catching up" on your sleep is by taking a nap in the mid-afternoon on the weekends. You may be thinking you don't have time to take naps in the afternoon, but there's much scientific validity for taking naps every day. As you may be aware, certain countries observe siestas, or short naps in the mid-afternoon. It's unlikely this will take hold in the US, but if you can find a way to do it, give it a try.

There are a number of scientific studies that tout the benefit of naps. I won't get into the details of all the studies, but in general, people who take naps are found to have a lower rate of cardiovascular disease. One recent study looked at over 23,000 Greek men and women, and found that working men who took frequent naps had a 64% lower risk of death from heart disease. Overall, the risk of dying from heart disease was 34% lower overall for people who took naps.

Not Too Little, Not Too Much

Another interesting issue that generates a lot of controversy is the ideal length of time one should sleep. There are some studies that show that not sleeping long enough is associated with increased risk of heart disease. One recent study reported that women who slept five hours per night had a 40% greater chance of having a heart attack than those who slept for eight hours. The interesting finding in this study, however, was that people who slept nine hours or more also had an increased risk of heart attack, although not as much compared with the sleep-deprived group.

This study suggests that although there may be an ideal number of hours one should sleep, it's different for every person. It's easy to conclude that sleeping for nine hours is unhealthy for your heart. But I'm willing to bet that if you took these same people who slept for nine hours and forced them to sleep for 6 to 7 hours, their risk of having a heart attack would increase even more. They have to sleep nine or more hours for a reason. This goes to show that it's an issue of poor quality, rather than poor quantity of sleep.

I have many patients who tell me that they are great sleepers. They claim to be able to sleep for 9 to 10 hours. However, many of these same people admit that they are still somewhat tired when they wake up and have trouble focusing or concentrating during the day. From a sleep-breathing perspective, this finding makes perfect sense. If you are not sleeping efficiently, then you'll try to make up for it by sleeping longer. But no matter how long you sleep, you'll never wake up refreshed.

There are also numerous people who sleep for only 5 to 6 hours every night and function well during the day. But if your 5 to 6 hours are of poor quality, then you won't be able to perform at peak capacity during the day, nor enjoy life outside of work. If this sounds like you, by all means, increase your total sleep time. Having a heart attack in ten years is not worth that promotion.

Avoid All Stimulants & Muscle Relaxants

There are also certain foods to avoid before bedtime. Anything that contains caffeine can have a stimulatory effect and should be avoided after 3 P.M. Alcohol not only irritates the stomach and aggravates acid reflux, but also has a relaxing effect on your muscles, including those of the throat. If you drink a night-cap, it may help you fall asleep faster, but alcohol is known to severely disrupt deep sleep. The combination of alcohol or any medication that relaxes the muscles and an anatomical predisposition to a sleep-breathing condition results in disrupted deep and REM sleep. Alcohol and caffeine can also be very dehydrating. Nicotine is also a well-known stimulant; therefore smoking before bedtime is counterproductive to a good night's sleep. This is in addition to the health risks of smoking in general. Nicotine also has been found to significantly relax the lower esophageal sphincter, promoting or aggravating acid reaching the throat. If you're still smoking and have failed nicotine replacement therapy, visit www.sleepinterrupted.com/quitstrugglefree.html to download or listen to a free audio on how to quit struggle free.

Stress Less and Breathe

Stress is a topic that's simple in concept, but difficult to control. In today's society, it's a fact of life. But I'm sure that you know of some people or certain cultures that seem to be oblivious to the fact that stress is even a word. But in our world, what can we do? I want to emphasize again that I'm not saying that stress causes a sleep-breathing condition, and vice versa, but that one can definitely aggravate the other.

The topic of stress management is beyond the scope of this book. There is, however, one technique in controlling stress that I have found helpful, which is the practice of breath control. The most sophisticated breathing techniques were developed in the yogic traditions. One in particular is pranayama, or the art of yoga breathing. Prana means life energy or life force, and yama means discipline or control, and ayama means expansion or extension. Various other cultures in the East have also developed their own method of breath control.

Breathing is something we take for granted. If you forget to do it, it's done automatically. If you're running, breathing speeds up, and when you're relaxed, it slows down. Breathing is unique in that it's under the control of both your voluntary and involuntary nervous systems. Your voluntary nervous system handles all the motor activities or other functions that are under your direct control. Your involuntary nervous system (or autonomic nervous system) controls your body functions automatically (breathing, heart rate, digestion, etc.), without you ever having to think about it. If you recall from previous chapters, it's broken down into two parts: the sympathetic (fight or flight), and the parasympathetic (rest and relaxation). Interestingly, the process of breathing in (inhalation) is controlled by your sympathetic nervous system, whereas breathing out (exhalation) is controlled by your parasympathetic nervous system. Using very sensitive electrical instruments, one can see the heart rate slowing down during exhalation and speeding up during inspiration. So when you breathe faster, your heart rate goes up. When you are nervous or angry, your breathing and heart rate also increase.

Many breathing experts agree that just being aware of your breathing will result in a slowing of the breath, thus lowering the heart rate and promoting stress reduction. Even better, slowing down the exhalation part relative to the inhalation part has a powerful effect on increasing your parasympathetic effects (or relaxation response), while reducing the sympathetic effects (stress response) of the autonomic nervous system. In effect, this technique can slow down your heart rate, and lower your stress levels. Musicians and professional speakers use these techniques to not only to relieve stress, but by breathing more deeply using the diaphragm rather than the upper chest, they are able to sing, play an instrument or speak more effectively. Experienced yoga practitioners would already be well versed in this phenomena.

I'm sure you've all heard someone say to you when you were nervous or stressed: "Take a slow, deep breath." Why did it work in most cases? Because of the effect of slowed breathing on your involuntary nervous system. This technique is even used in sex therapy for premature ejaculation. The man is instructed to take slow, deep breaths, which calms the sympathetic nervous system (which controls ejaculation). If you're also stressed about your performance in bed, then the sympathetic nervous system can overwhelm the parasympathetic nervous system, which normally causes an erection. This can lead to either erectile dysfunction, or premature ejaculation. The same nervous system principles apply to women as well.

One simple breathing technique that is taught by Dr. Andrew Weil, noted integrative medicine expert, is the "relaxing breath." If performed regularly, at least twice daily, its cumulative effects on your well-being can be dramatic. Sit in a comfortable position with your back straight and your head upright, and your hands on your legs. Pay attention to your breathing by focusing on your breath as you breathe in and out. Spend time watching the breath, trying to breathe quieter, slower, deeper and more regularly than you normally would. Make sure to breathe in using your diaphragm, so that your abdomen protrudes with each inhalation. Take a slow in-breath counting to four, pause to a count of seven and then breathe slowly outwards to a count of eight. Repeat this four times. You may have to practice at first to adhere to this counting regime. Do not force, just slowly work towards the 4–7–8 pattern. These four breath cycles can be performed when in a stressful situation, while driving, or before going to bed. This powerful technique helps to calm the stress state and can be used to control anxiety or other stress-related conditions.

These short breathing "pauses" can also help you transition from one major task to another throughout the day.

There are so many good books and audio programs on breathing available, so I can't make a recommendation. Choose one that you can commit to on a regular basis. You can read a book, listen to a CD, or take yoga courses. Whatever it is, focus specifically on breathing techniques that promote relaxation.

Try Acupuncture

Acupuncture is another way of altering your overactive stress response. It's widely published that acupuncture does modify your nerve pathways, rebalancing and bringing into line the overactive sympathetic nervous system. Interestingly, a recent study looked at using acupuncture for people with mild to moderate OSA. They showed that the AHI dropped about 50% on average after multiple sessions.[1]

So regardless of what relaxes you, whether it's breathing exercises, yoga, reading a book, or physical exercise, make it a point to incorporate a routine into your daily schedule. It may not cure your sleep-breathing problem, but it could potentially lessen how your body responds to the sleep-breathing condition, lowering your stress levels, and allowing you to cope better with life despite not sleeping as well as you could be.

Some of you may already be doing many of the things that I just mentioned, because you find that it helps you to feel better. Now you know why you started doing these things in the first place.

Tips for Insomnia and Better Sleep Hygiene

It's not uncommon for people with sleep-breathing conditions to also suffer from insomnia. I've described my paradigm's viewpoint on insomnia in a previous chapter. It's only natural that multiple arousals from partial or complete throat collapse can lead to a heightened awake response, increasing your stress levels as well. Whether you can't fall asleep or keep waking up after you've fallen asleep, once it starts, it turns into a vicious cycle. The stress and anxiety over worrying about not being able to sleep increases the "awake" response, further aggravating the insomnia. There are a number of reasons for insomnia, one of which is sleep-breathing related, but if you have any other cause, the arousals caused by the sleep-breathing condition just aggravate whatever other problems you may have.

Here are some general recommendations for people with insomnia. Try to develop a routine before going to bed, or do something relaxing for 30 to 60 minutes before bedtime. Taking a hot shower or bath or reading a book just before going to sleep, will remind you that you are about to go to sleep. Make sure you take your shower or bath about one hour before you plan on going to bed. The hot water temperature raises your body temperature, and as your body temperature begins to drop an hour later, you'll feel sleepy. Since you want to promote a drop in your body temperature, making your room relatively colder will help you fall asleep more easily as well.

Use your bed only for sleep and sex. Don't read, eat, watch TV or talk on the phone in bed.

Make sure your room is sufficiently dark when you are about to go to bed. It seems that the newer LED lights in current electronics are much brighter these days. With only three or four devices, my entire bedroom was lit up to the point where I could see everything in the room. I had to resort to placing black electrical tape over each LED. Make sure your windows are fully covered and dark enough so that sunlight does not shine through in the morning. If this is not adequate, use an eye mask. Remember, light blocks melatonin production, which can only start to rise in total darkness.

If you can't fall asleep after 15 to 30 minutes, get out of bed and sit quietly for 15 to 30 minutes. Practice your relaxing breathing exercises or read a boring book, and then go back to sleep when you begin to feel drowsy. It's better to read a book and go to sleep 30 minutes later than to toss and turn in your bed for 1 to 2 hours. If the same thing happens again, you may want to go to bed thirty minutes later than your normal sleep time. Keep going to bed later and later until your total sleep time matches your total time in bed, then gradually increase your total sleep time back up to 7 to 8 hours. Also, don't take naps during the day if you're going through this process.

Snacks high in tryptophan are traditionally recommended for insomnia (such as turkey, bananas, dates, or warm milk). But again, if you have a sleep-breathing issue, although you may fall asleep faster, you may wake up more frequently in the night.

There are a number of alternatives to counting sheep; I will mention a handful for the sake of completeness. I'm sure there are hundreds of other methods that I'm missing. If you have an important presentation in the morning and you can't sleep because you're stressed, instead of saying to yourself, "I have to get some sleep or I'm going to embarrass myself tomorrow," say it much slower to yourself, like a tape recorder in slow speed. Stretch out each word, syllable and letter and make it as slow as possible. This diverts your attention from worrying about your presentation to manipulating the sounds instead. Some people visually write all their problems on a chalkboard and erase each problem, one by one. If you toss and turn, instead of quick, jerking movements, do it in slow motion, take a deep slow breath, smile, and say to yourself, "I allow myself to fall asleep." You can also try the relaxing breath exercise that was described earlier in this chapter.

Sleep Promoting Supplements

Many integrative medicine and herbal experts, as well as many of my own patients, swear by valerian. It's from the root of a perennial herb commonly found in North America, and can be found in health food stores and comes in various strengths. It should be taken about 1 to 2 hours before bedtime, and works better if you take it regularly, rather than on nights that you can't sleep. It also has a mild sedative, anti-anxiety property, with no significant drowsiness or side effects during the day.

Melatonin is also available in common health food stores. Try to purchase the synthetic, or pharmacy grade, version since "natural" melatonin comes from animal brains and can harbor viruses or cause allergic reactions. It should be taken 30 to 60 minutes before bedtime. Even though this is sold over the counter, it's still a hormone, and you should talk to your doctor before taking melatonin. Melatonin is also useful for jet-lag and sleep-wake timing disorders.

Cognitive Behavioral Therapy

Cognitive behavioral therapy (CBT) has been shown to help many people battle insomnia. It helps to retrain your negative thoughts about sleep into positive ones. Best results are achieved under the guidance of a health care professional, but there are various versions available to the lay public in multiple formats such as books, CDs and audiotapes. CBT was found to be effective in 75 to 80% of people with chronic insomnia, and was also found more effective than sleeping pills. If the above conservative measures don't work for you, then find out about CBT in your area, or look online (one option is www.sleepcoach.net).

Sleeping Pills

Sleeping pills are used by many people to deal with their sleep problems, regardless of what's causing the problem. With advances in modern medicine, there are a number of "safer" sleep aids that are on the market, as evidenced by a myriad of TV commercials on the air. I'm not saying you should never take sleeping pills, but you should try to avoid them as much as possible. They should be used only as a last resort. If you are considering using them, take a look at what you can do to change your behavior during the day, so that you can taper off the pill only after a few doses. The newest medications last only for a few hours with no drowsiness in the morning, but they all can have various side effects. Some of the older-type sleeping pills are used for their other properties, such as an antidepressant for people with insomnia and depression. Remember that any medication, if it relaxes the throat structures, can aggravate underlying sleep-breathing problems. Many people mistakenly take sleeping pills thinking they have insomnia when in fact they have OSA.

Get a full medical exam to ensure there's no treatable medical problem, and consult your doctor about your sleep problems. A good physician should ask more specific questions about the nature of your sleep problem. If he or she is too quick to give you a prescription, be wary—either the doctor is too time constrained to have a more thorough discussion with you, or the doctor was not properly trained in these issues.

Ideally, you shouldn't have to take a pill at all, whether it's a prescription sleeping pill or a natural herbal pill. You should try to take advantage of your body's natural inner sleep clock to achieve deep and restorative sleep. Ultimately, it's more important to focus on changing what you do when you are *awake*, rather than to focus on what you can do to fall asleep. But when you do try a pill, use it with caution and make every effort to wean yourself off it as soon as possible, while making an effort to follow the conservative recommendations in this chapter.

24 Feeling Better with Medical Intervention

A FTER YOU HAVE EXHAUSTED ALL conservative options, and once you have been officially diagnosed with OSA, there are two basic non-surgical ways of treating your sleep-breathing problem. One way is to use continuous positive airway pressure, or a CPAP machine, and the other way is to pull your lower jaw forward at night while sleeping using a mandibular advancement device (MAD). This also applies to people with upper airway resistance syndrome (UARS). Surgical management will be discussed in the next chapter.

Using CPAP

For most people CPAP is the first line of treatment. It involves placing a mask over your nose to blow mild positive air pressure through your breathing passageways to keep your throat tissues from collapsing at night. Not a very pleasant thought, but effective, in theory. For many people who are able to use it, it's a life-saver, with spectacular results. Others, however, absolutely refuse to use it.

Once a diagnosis of significant OSA is confirmed, your doctor will present the option of undergoing a CPAP titration study, where you go through the same sleep study process again, but this time, a mask is placed securely over your face. As you sleep, the air pressure is gradually adjusted upwards until the best level is reached, confirming that your breathing pauses are almost or completely gone. Most people don't feel any better after the titration study, but there are some who are amazed how well they slept even on a few hours of good deep sleep at the optimal pressure. A CPAP machine is then ordered for your home and adjusted to this pressure setting.

A technician from the respiratory equipment company will set it up for you and show you how to use it. This can happen either at home or in the company's offices. They will also check up on you to make sure that you are adjusting to the machine and answer any questions that you may have. One word of caution: The quality of customer service by your equipment company varies significantly from inadequate to excellent. Take a pro-active approach. If you don't hear from anyone or if there is a problem, call the company and give them your feedback. There are tens of thousands of people going through similar situations, and there are solutions and answers for almost every problem imaginable.

You can also call your sleep lab or doctor involved in your care. Don't feel guilty about calling, or feel like you're being a pain. One of my greatest frustrations is that follow-up with patients starting on CPAP is poor in general, especially when you have to deal with two or three different parties for one condition. It's been shown time and again that good support and follow-up is critical to high success rates for people using and actually benefiting from CPAP.

CPAP works well in patients who use it. The problem is that many patients don't use it for various reasons. Some just don't like having something strapped to their face, some can't move around in bed, and others may feel claustrophobic. If your nose is stuffy, the pressure needs to be higher and ends up irritating your nose. This problem can be readily addressed, as described in Chapter 20.

CPAP compliance statistics vary anywhere from around 40 to 80%. Compliance can mean different things. One typical definition defined compliance as using the machine for at least four hours per night. It seems that since there is no standard definition of compliance, everyone uses a different standard, leading to a wide range of numbers.

Unfortunately, from what I have seen, the overall long-term compliance is dismal—in the 10–20% range. My guess if that if you are involved in a research study looking at compliance, you'll be more likely to use CPAP. But in the real world, compliance numbers just can't come close to matching numbers under controlled research conditions. The more follow-up and support there is (especially in the first few weeks), the higher the chance that the person will use CPAP and gain significant benefit from using it. Studies have also proven this. The problem is that counseling and follow-up is very time and labor intensive, something that very few doctors and equipment suppliers are able to offer.

Despite the grim statistics, I strongly recommend a CPAP trial for anyone who has significant OSA. If you don't like it, then at least you know you can't use it and can move on to other options. If you have UARS, this is also an option. Based on Dr. Guilleminault's original research study describing UARS, the majority of people did well at a relatively low pressure setting. I have a handful of UARS patients who find CPAP helpful, but the vast majority cannot tolerate using it, particularly because they are usually light sleepers and are very easily aroused by any form of stimulation, especially masks or devices on their faces.

Many studies have also shown that people with very low levels of OSA can't use or benefit from CPAP very well, whereas patients with severe OSA tend to do much better. I see this as well in my practice. Older people tend to accept it more widely, but young single men and especially women are usually resistant to using CPAP at night. You can probably guess why this is so.

In my experience, about 25% of people who undergo CPAP titration have a very positive experience, another 25% absolutely hate it, and the remaining 50% have mixed results. The 25% who dislike it refuse to try it at home, and then this is when we begin talking about other options. With the remainder I strongly recommend that they try

CPAP at home on a trial basis, of which, roughly half end up using CPAP on a long-term basis, and later tapering down to much lower levels. Unfortunately, many people stop using CPAP altogether and never follow-up.

Some of the more common problems I see people have using CPAP include a mask leak, mouth leak, too much pressure when exhaling, and taking the mask off unknowingly. If the mask is not properly fitted or of the wrong size, there can be an air leak which can blow air into your eyes or make noises. This is easily corrected by adjusting the mask or headgear, or replacing the mask with a different model. An alternative to a nasal mask is what's called "nasal pillows": Instead of a mask over your nose, a thin tube runs across your upper lip with two soft prongs that fit into your nostrils from below. If you are interested in what these masks look like, just search "CPAP" in your web browser and you'll see many different options.

If you leak air through your mouth, then not only will you feel it and wake up, but the pressure that enters your windpipe will be lower and your CPAP will not work. One remedy is to use a chin strap that keeps your mouth closed. Or, you can try a full-face mask, which goes over your mouth and nose. It is a little more uncomfortable than standard nasal masks or pillows, but for some, it makes a big difference. There are literally dozens of options to choose from, so if one doesn't work, keep trying other masks. An alternative "mask," called CPAP Pro, is a hybrid nasal "pillow" that is attached to a dental device which is custom fitted onto your teeth. Some of my patients like it. It can be found at www.cpappro.com.

One valuable online resource to look at is www.cpaptalk.com. It's run by cpap.com, which is an online CPAP equipment retailer. A basic CPAP machine starts around $250. Masks start around $50. Most insurances will cover for CPAP machines if you have OSA. There are a number of educational videos, articles and useful resources on this site, along with an active user forum. Look under "Our Collective Wisdom" for a great list of topics to read on everything related to CPAP. Use the forum to post your questions. You should take everything on the internet with a grain of salt, but there can be a pearl or two found on this site. You can even browse the online store to see what equipment options are available. Please note that I don't have any financial interest in this company. I just find it to be a useful resource to help you navigate the confusing and apprehensive feelings that can go along with being a first-time CPAP user.

Another useful site for anyone with sleep problems is www. talkaboutsleep.com. It's a very active forum and discussion group, with some very vocal participants, but useful if you know where to look or ask the right questions. The American Sleep Apnea Association also has a great sleep apnea support forum (www. apneasupport.org).

There are a dizzying number of options, features and upgrades when choosing a CPAP machine. Some people will tout advantages with Bi-PAP (bilevel PAP), or Auto-PAP, but in general, unless there is an unusual situation, most people do very well with a basic CPAP machine.

For people who feel that they can't exhale because the pressure is too high, there are two options: Bi-PAP which automatically lowers the pressure during exhalation to a predetermined level, or computer algorithm-generated pressure changes (one type is C-Flex™), which gradually lowers the pressure during exhalation, rather than an abrupt drop that occurs in Bi-PAP.

If you find yourself pulling off your mask in the middle of the night without even knowing it, then you may need to talk to your sleep doctor or equipment supplier about trying another mask or headgear. Unfortunately, this is one of the most common situations that predict not being able to use the mask long-term.

Just because you start CPAP does not mean that you are committed for life. You can always choose one of the other options, if you are a good candidate. If you have mild sleep apnea, and have some weight to lose, losing that weight can lower your AHI number to the point where you may not need CPAP anymore. In theory, sleeping better can facilitate weight loss through more exercise and improved metabolism. If you have severe OSA, however, it's less likely you can come off CPAP, even with significant weight loss.

Mandibular Advancement Device

Mandibular advancement devices (MAD) are another good option for people with OSA, snoring, and UARS, especially if the major reason for obstruction comes from tongue collapse. If so, a consultation with a dentist who specializes in this area is recommended. If you sleep much better on your side or stomach, rather than your back, and you do not have enlarged tonsils, you may be a good candidate. One way of confirming this is to see an ear, nose and throat specialist who can look at your tongue position with a camera while on your back. Dentists have their own way of measuring this as well, including physical examination and x-rays.

A mandibular advancement device basically involves the creation of a mold that is made of your upper and lower teeth, which is then sent to a laboratory. A prosthesis is custom made and sent back for fitting and adjustment. The bottom part of the device (attached to your lower jaw) can be adjusted so that it slides outwards, little by little, on a weekly or monthly basis. This gradual advancement allows for better tolerance and less discomfort. It is continuously adjusted forward until you either don't snore anymore, sleep improves and you wake feeling more refreshed. If it gets pulled too far, you'll feel pain or discomfort in your jaw or teeth. At this point, the lower part is pushed back and set to its previous comfortable position.

If you go this route, and you get to a point where your sleep has improved significantly, it's very important that a repeat sleep study is performed to confirm that the apneas and hypopneas are significantly improved. It's unreasonable to expect your numbers to go down to zero or the low single digits (unlike CPAP). A significant drop in a range under 10 is usually acceptable. So if your AHI is 30, then a drop to seven is considered acceptable, as long as you are feeling much better. If you have UARS or very mild OSA, then the numbers don't matter as much since you're starting from a relatively low number to begin with—what's more important is how you feel.

Similar to CPAP, success and tolerance with MADs varies widely. Initial success (with various definitions) can go up as high as 70–80%. Most studies reported better success in patient with mild to moderate

OSA, compared with patients with severe OSA. In general, it works very well for snoring. However, a one year follow-up study reported that 55% were still using their devices, while only 37% of people were still using it every night. Reasons for stopping included pain and discomfort and lack of effectiveness. While I have seen many patients benefit greatly from MADs, I've also seen a significant drop-off in use over time.

Regardless, you won't know whether or not you'll like it, and more importantly, if it will work for you, until you try. Some of you may have already used a splint for TMJ or dental grinding. If you can tolerate a splint, then a MAD may work for you. If you can't tolerate a TMJ device, you may not be a good candidate for a MAD for two reasons: it may aggravate TMJ, or you just can't sleep with something inside your mouth. Side effects include dry mouth, discomfort, TMJ aggravation, or bite changes. If you have multiple missing teeth, or have multiple caps or crowns, then you're probably not an ideal candidate. I'm told by dentists that MADs don't cause TMJ, rather it can help people with TMJ. Everyone is different, so check with a dental specialist regarding these issues for a full consultation to see if you are a possible candidate. You can also find out about the process, what to expect, price, etc. Your insurance may or may not cover you for these devices so it's wise to check with your insurance company first. Costs can vary from just under $1000 to well over $2000, depending on the model.

A less expensive "screening test" that I sometimes recommend is to order a simple anti-snoring device over the internet (www.nosnorezone.com and www.sleeppro.com). There are a number of "boil-and-bite" MADs available, which cost from $55 to $300. These are plastic splints that are softened by placing in boiling water and then biting down on them with your lower jaw thrust forward. It's a low-tech version of a MAD, and not readily adjustable. I usually recommend starting with the lowest priced model and trying it with two goals: Does it help with sleep quality, and can you keep it in your mouth without significant discomfort? If the answer is yes to both, it may be worthwhile investing in a formal, adjustable MAD.

25 Feeling Better with Surgery

BEFORE I TALK ABOUT SURGICAL OPTIONS, I'd like to mention an interesting phenomenon amongst many of my patients who undergo sleep apnea surgery. For the most part, the way a patient feels after surgery correlates well with objective measures as seen on a sleep study that's performed 6 to 12 months after the surgery. However, there are two small groups of patients that seem to have paradoxical results. For instance, the first group has excellent results according to the post-operative sleep study, where the number of breathing pauses drop from 60 to 10 times per hour. However, they do not feel any significant improvement in the quality of their sleep. The second group, on the other hand, has the reverse effect: The number may not drop very much at all, but they feel significantly better. There are a lot of possible technical explanations for these situations, but there's one other reason that I think is worth discussing.

Dr. Maxwell Maltz, a plastic surgeon in the 1950s, describes in his book, *Psycho-Cybernetics*, an interesting phenomenon where some of his patients' perception of their results was dramatically out of line with the actual surgical results. For example, certain patients undergoing rhinoplasty would be ecstatic about the results, even if the changes were very minor. Others who experienced more dramatic improvements in their facial appearance, still refused to believe that there was any improvement.

I've personally seen a similar situation occur when I was a resident in training. While opening up a checking account at my local bank branch, the accounts associate, when he found out that I was an ear, nose and throat surgeon, told me that he was not happy with the shape of his nose. Since I was just a resident, I referred him to one of my professors who specialized in facial plastic surgery. The procedure went well, and many months later when I saw him again, he seemed much happier and told me that he'd just been promoted. Over the next few months to years, he continued to receive multiple promotions, and was eventually recruited to another bank for much higher pay, with many more responsibilities.

What the above examples show is that you can perform the same surgery on five different patients, and get five vastly different results, whether it's in the rate of complications, or in the patient's subjective or objective sense of improvement. What I find to be a crucial component in how patients perceive whether or not their surgery was a success is their pre-surgery state of mind. In general, people who do well don't look to the surgery as the ultimate solution to their problems— rather, they view their surgery as one component of many changes they must now undertake to improve their health and well being.

The surgery is not meant to be a "cure" for their problems, but a substantial boost in a process to help patients to feel well enough so that they can have the energy and motivation to continue and take over on their own. Ultimately, the patients that are most satisfied with the results are the ones most likely to see the surgery as a starting point to make major life changes in how they eat, exercise, or even in how they deal with stress. For people who are overweight, losing 5 to 15 pounds helps this process along as well.

When the patient and I decide together to proceed with surgery, I see it as a life-long relationship, rather than a one-time fix. Over the years, the forces that promote upper airway narrowing may creep in, or there may be other minor issues that need to be addressed. Some people don't get the results that they want, and only through open dialogue and trust can further progress be made.

Surgery is not for everyone. If you're not sure about surgery, take your time, do your research, and talk to other patients who have undergone similar procedures. This is purely elective surgery, so you don't absolutely *have* to undergo the procedure. The challenge for both the patient and the surgeon is knowing if and when surgery should take place at all. For many of those who go on to take the leap, the results can be dramatically life-changing. With all this in mind, I will now address surgical treatment options for OSA, upper airway resistance syndrome, and other sleep-related breathing disorders.

Does Surgery Work?

There is much confusion about snoring and sleep apnea procedures. Some people say that surgery should never be done because the uvulopalatopharyngoplasty (UPPP) procedure, involving removal of palatal soft tissue, doesn't work. Based on large-scale published studies,[1] and in my own experience, the success rate is about 40%. We now know that the palate is not the only area that requires attention, and once you address all the areas appropriately, success rates can be much higher. The real challenge is in selecting the right patient to offer UPPP surgery. Skeptics should try arguing their case with the 40% of people who are happy with their surgical results.

I have to admit that being a surgeon, I have a biased view on this subject. It's truly gratifying to see patients' lives transformed after sleep apnea surgery. It's equally frustrating that I can't help many more people who are not good candidates for surgery. The same frustration applies to a minority of patients who undergo major surgical procedures yet don't improve at all. But long ago, I decided that my surgical services were valuable as an alternative to CPAP and mandibular advancement devices, and as long as the patient has realistic expectations, surgery is a worthwhile process.

As I discussed in previous chapters, one major reason for the development of OSA and UARS is due to narrowed mouth and throat anatomy. This can lead to hormonal, neurologic, and physiologic changes, which can then feed back to worsen OSA, resulting in a vicious cycle. Why then bother with invasive surgery treating only one part of this complex process with no guarantee of success? My answer is that it depends on the reason for and the type of surgery that is undertaken. The more aggressive and appropriate the surgery, the higher the success rate. The key is to tailor the type and appropriateness of the procedures to the patient's anatomy, with a full understanding of why we're doing the procedures and what to expect. In an ideal scenario, the anatomic area of obstruction is definitively addressed, and the sleep-breathing problem is resolved.

The following is a clear-cut example of the benefits of surgery over more conservative measures under the right circumstances. Let's suppose that you have a small bead stuck in one of your windpipes that's been causing a chronic cough for months. One option is to control the cough with medications, or give antibiotics for a presumed bronchitis. All these conservative, non-invasive options do help control your cough, but it never "cures" the problem. The bead causes an anatomic obstruction, and needs to be dealt with structurally—it should be physically removed. No amount of anti-cough, anti-inflammatory, antibiotic medications will ever solve this problem. In a similar way, sleep-breathing problems are essentially an anatomic problem, and should be treated as such, with the caveat that some people respond better to structural changes than others.

Up until the early 1980s, when CPAP was developed, the only option for OSA treatment was a tracheotomy. This is a procedure where a surgical hole is made in the windpipe, just below the voice box. Although this procedure has a 100% success rate, it's not a very practical solution, since you have to breathe through a small tube in your throat, and have to clean and take care of both the opening in your neck and the tubing as well. All other surgical options compared to a tracheotomy are less than perfect, but still worthwhile in certain carefully selected patients.

Coincidentally, the UPPP procedure was first presented to the public in the early 1980s as well. Initial UPPP success rates were good, but with time, the success rate dropped to about 40%, which is the standard quoted success rate. This is where all the confusion starts. People (physicians and patients) began to state that a UPPP procedure does *not work*, whereas CPAP *works all the time*. However, this is like comparing apples to oranges.

Although CPAP does treat OSA effectively, as I stated previously, not many people are able to take advantage of it. And of those who are able to use it, not everyone continues to use it indefinitely. The UPPP procedure, on the other hand, does work in about 40% of patients, but only in those people whose main area of airway narrowing comes from the soft palate and tonsil area. UPPP therefore does not work, or works only partially, on the vast majority of patients with OSA, since most have some or a significant degree of tongue collapse as well.

But let's say that out of 100 people with OSA, 40%, or 40 people would be considered "cured" after UPPP. One definition of surgical success is that the number of breathing pauses (greater than 10 seconds) per hour (or the apnea hypopnea index, or AHI) after surgery has to be less than 20 every hour and overall drop more than 50% of the pre-surgical number of pauses. Of course, there will be many other people with partial improvements, but not official "cures." Compare the above group with 100 people who are placed on CPAP, and let's say optimistically 60% of those people are able to use CPAP successfully every night. That means there is a 60% "success" rate. But over time, many people will stop using it. Let's say that conservatively one third of the people who started using CPAP stopped after a few months or years. This leaves us with a 40% overall success rate, which is equivalent to the UPPP group.

An interesting study performed at a Veteran's Administration hospital center revealed similar findings. They looked at patients who were diagnosed with OSA between 1997 and 2001.[2] By 2001, patients who underwent UPPP were more likely to be alive than patients placed on CPAP, but only by a small margin. What the authors of this study imply is that even though only about 40% of people who underwent

UPPP were adequately treated, UPPP actually outperforms CPAP in terms of absolute survival rates. The reason for this finding is that once you undergo a successful surgical procedure, you have a 100% compliance rate, whereas CPAP patients slowly drop off the rate at which they use their machines.

There are other valid criticisms with the UPPP procedure: In many cases, "cured" patients still have low levels of OSA which are considered unacceptable if one was using CPAP. Sometimes after UPPP, the sleep apnea condition worsens. There are other various reasons against undergoing surgery such as anesthesia complications, the pain and discomfort involved, or a permanent leakage of air or fluid into the nose when swallowing. Regardless, which would you choose: a 1% chance of nasal regurgitation (which can be treated), or a 3–5 times increased risk of heart attack or stroke? As you can see, it's all relative.

I'm not promoting surgery over CPAP by any means. I'm trying to bring to discussion the pros and cons of both options, pointing out that there's no clear obvious advantage for either side. Conservative options should always be tried first, but surgical options should never be ruled out, especially if you don't know the facts behind these other options. Unfortunately, many patients are never offered a consultation to determine their potential for successful surgery. Even when they do undergo surgery, many patients undergo the UPPP procedure alone without proper evaluation of other areas that can aggravate palatal collapse (tongue or nose), thus leading to the low 40% success figure.

Going Beyond the Palate

Once you go beyond the palate, the picture looks much better for surgery. I mentioned previously that a tracheotomy is almost 100% effective for treating OSA. Everything else you do above the voice box is not as good, but acceptable. The next most successful operation is the maxillo-mandibular advancement or MMA, where maxillofacial surgeons physically cut and move the upper and lower

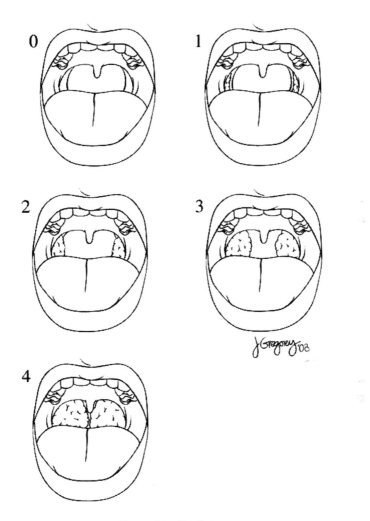

Figure 25.1 Tonsil size.

jaws forward. This opens the airway behind the palate and tongue. It works anywhere from 90–95% of the time. Even then, there's still a few percent chance that after going through this extensive surgery, you may not get the results that you want.

Initial work by doctors affiliated with Stanford has shown that if you address all the areas of the upper airway that can potentially collapse (nose, palate, tongue), then the success rate can be as high

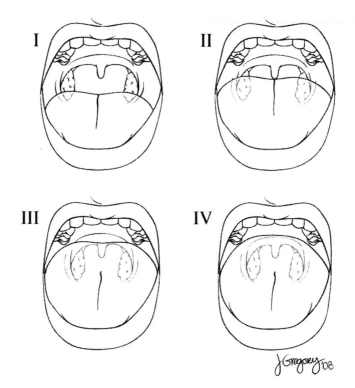

Figure 25.2 Tongue position. Notice that the higher the tongue position, due to narrower jaw width, the narrower the oropharyngeal space, with the tonsils appearing closer together.

as about 75%.[3] This is a significant improvement over the 40% figure cited previously. The main reason for this significant improvement is the addition of procedures that address tongue and voice box collapse. The nose is addressed as well. This is called multi-level site-directed surgery. It makes sense: open up all the areas that can obstruct breathing. Of the remaining 20% who fail these procedures, going on to MMA worked very well for most of these people.

One useful way of determining whether or not you may be a good candidate for UPPP surgery alone is to apply the Friedman classification.[4] In brief, Dr. Friedman states that if you have very large tonsils (tonsil size 3 or 4; Figure 25.1), and you can see your tonsils and the lower free edge of your soft palate just behind your tongue (tongue position I or II; Figure 25.2), and your body mass index (kg/m^2) is under 40, then your chances of success is about 80%. Anything else is in the unfavorable group (small or no tonsils or a high sitting tongue), and your chances of success are about 40% or lower. In these situations, additional tongue or hyoid procedures are probably needed. Just like any other questionnaire, you have to take it with a grain of salt and look at it in light of the whole person (i.e., other anatomical factors, lifestyle, expectations, etc.). You should never use this tool alone to determine candidacy for a surgical procedure.

Addressing the Palate

In determining the various procedures available to effectively improve breathing efficiency, it's important to address all the different types of procedures that are applicable to the palate. Most people with palate level obstruction will need some type of palatal surgery, whether it's a simple stiffening (injection snoreplasty or Pillar implants; see Appendix A) or the standard UPPP procedure. There are also a number of variations of the basic UPPP procedure. One lesser invasive alternative called the uvulo-palatal flap involves removing only the mucous membrane layer covering the soft palate muscle and stitching the raw surfaces closed. Because no muscle needs to be cut, in theory, it's much less painful.

There are probably another dozen or so variations of the UPPP. The key point is that regardless of which procedure your surgeon recommends, needless to say, it must be done well. If the surgeon is too conservative for fear of causing complications, then he or she has done you a disservice. If too aggressive, then that's a problem too. In general, it's probably wiser to be too conservative than too aggressive, since it's harder to replace lost tissue. Additional tissue can always be removed in a subsequent procedure if necessary.

Everyone's anatomy is different, but for most people, a basic UPPP procedure, done well, should be adequate in controlling palatal narrowing and snoring. For those people with unusual anatomy, the surgeon must tailor the procedure to the patient's unique throat structures.

One technical change that I incorporated many years ago involves using a "Coblation" wand to perform the tonsillectomy and make cuts on the soft palate. The Coblation® wand is a handheld device that vaporizes soft tissue at relatively low temperatures. I use it routinely for tonsillectomies and I find that it cuts down on pain and discomfort significantly. Since using it as a cutting tool, rather than using electrocautery (which cuts and chars tissues at high temperatures), my UPPP patients have experienced significantly less pain after this procedure and are able to return home earlier.

Addressing Tongue Collapse

There are a number of different ways of addressing the problem of tongue collapse. You can think of these surgical methods as a permanent way of pulling the base of the tongue forward, without moving your entire jaw forward. Some are very aggressive, and others are minimally invasive. Procedures range from shrinking or physically modifying the tongue base, or pulling the tongue base forward, to pulling the hyoid bone down or forward. This is done without making any major modifications to the facial bony skeleton.

One of the more aggressive tongue reduction procedures is called a partial glossectomy. In essence, a wedge-shaped portion is cut from the base of the tongue. There are many variations to this procedure, but due to pain and possible bleeding issues, it's not done very often anymore, especially when there are lesser invasive and equally effective methods available.

A more recent tongue "shrinking" procedure involves placing a thin needle into the back of the tongue muscles and applying a measured amount of radiofrequency energy, which causes thermal damage, or a slight burn. Over time, as the tissue heals, a scar reaction occurs, which tightens and shrinks the tongue to a limited degree. This is why these procedures need to be repeated multiple times. Typically, the first procedure is performed along with a UPPP in the operating room, but another three to four treatments are needed in the office, about one month apart. Unfortunately, many people find it hard to finish all the required treatments, and are unable to obtain the full potential benefits of this procedure. Published studies on this subject express similar findings.

One variation of the above procedure involves placing the Coblation® wand through a small tunnel to the back of the tongue and vaporizing the muscular tissues in the actual base of the tongue.[5] Because it coagulates and vaporizes simultaneously, there is little bleeding, and only one session is needed. Dr. Eric Maier reported using this procedure on children with abnormally large tongues accompanied by associated breathing difficulties, and met with good results. Long-term results on adults undergoing this procedure are not yet available.

One of the more common procedures that is used for tongue base collapse is mandibular osteotomy with genioglossus advancement, or MOGA. In this procedure, a small rectangular portion of bone is cut from the lower midline bottom section of the jawbone, which is then advanced forward, pulling with it the attached genioglossus and geniohyoid muscles. Its location is kept in place using a screw. Although relatively safe and effective in experienced hands, risks include numbness of the lips, dental pain, tooth injury, or jaw fracture.

A lesser invasive but similarly effective procedure is to loop a thin nylon thread around the back of the tongue and attach it to the back of the midline jawbone. The purpose is to suspend the tongue, not pull it forward. In this way the tongue does not fall back during deep sleep, especially while on your back.

Another additional procedure that is commonly performed in addition to the above is what's called a hyoid myotomy with suspension (HMS). The hyoid bone is a c-shaped bone just above your voice box, which supports various tongue and voice box structures. If pulled forward, the base of the tongue and the top of the voice box also move forward, thus opening up the space behind the tongue. This procedure alone was found to lower the AHI in sleep apnea patients by about 50%.[6]

Many other published studies show that the combination of a UPPP, hyoid myotomy with suspension, and either a genioglossus advancement or tongue base radiofrequency procedure has around a 75–80% success rate.[7-9] It could be better, but it's double the overall success rate of a UPPP alone. This includes the suture suspension procedure and the tongue base radiofrequency procedures as well. People who don't respond to these procedures can opt for the maxillo-mandibular advancement procedure. Rarely, the palatal procedure or the tongue procedure may need to be repeated.

One last innovative procedure of note, especially for children, is palatal distraction therapy. Children have much more malleable bones, so changing the shape and appearance of the upper jaw is much simpler than with adults. In this procedure, an orthodontic device is placed on the upper jaw between the molars to gradually push the teeth apart, thus widening the upper jaw bone.

There are also situations where the lower jaw is so small in some infants, that without immediate surgical intervention, death is inevitable without a tracheotomy. There are a number of various congenital conditions where the jaw is severely underformed, which is potentially life-threatening. The procedure used, called distraction osteogenesis, involves a cut being made through the hard outer corti-cal bone on both sides of the jaw. Screws are placed on either side of the cuts, and attached to a thin rod either outside the skin or inside the mouth. A screw on the inserted rod is turned a predetermined amount on a weekly or biweekly basis so that the pins push apart from each other thus widening the jaw structure. The soft part of the inner bone can readily accommodate stretching and once set at the new length, hard outer cortical bone forms around the stretched inner part. Within a few months, the jaw lengthens and not only does the jaw look relatively normal, but the tracheotomy tube can be removed. I have to admit I was truly amazed when I first saw the before and after pictures of these infants and toddlers. Although not very appli-cable to adults at this point (because our bones are less flexible and more difficult to manipulate), I have seen sporadic case reports of this procedure being performed in normal adults for OSA.

When All is Said and Done

In general, if you are severely overweight (Body Mass Index or BMI > 40), then your chances of success with surgery are not as good as someone with a relatively low BMI. In this scenario, if you have no other options, one of the weight loss surgical procedures may improve your sleep apnea significantly. There is also the possibility that even if the surgery is initially successful, over time OSA symptoms may slowly return, especially as one ages or gains weight.

For people who don't officially meet the criteria for OSA, such as in UARS patients, surgery for any obvious area of obstruction could improve their quality of life dramatically. If you do undergo any form of sleep-breathing surgery, it's important to follow-up and undergo a sleep study about 4 to 6 months after the procedure. Even if you feel better, an objective measurement at the sleep center is important to know.

Not everyone will want surgery, even if it's a good option. And many people who want surgery will not be good candidates. Prior to surgery, you should consider what all the risks are, as well as look into all the various alternatives to surgery. Sleep-breathing surgery must be tailored to the individual's unique anatomy, so there's no one procedure that's appropriate for everyone.

I can't emphasize enough how much every person has different needs and priorities, and this is why developing a productive, fruitful relationship with your surgeon is crucial in determining the ultimate outcome. I truly believe that a good relationship between a surgeon and patient, as well the patient's healthy mindset is ultimately more important in determining the final outcome than my technical expertise as a surgeon.

26 Conclusion: Your Inspiration for Better Health

Life is really simple, but we insist on making it complicated.
— Confucius

I F YOU THINK ABOUT IT, the entire sleep-breathing paradigm may seem too simple of an explanation for all the complex medical conditions from which we human suffer. In this age of gene therapy, stereotactic radiosurgery and research on dozens of various inflammatory mediators, a simple breathing problem at night is a hard pill to swallow to explain many of your various ailments, especially when there are more sophisticated and exotic names to choose from.

All the individual concepts and disease processes I've described in this book are not new. Everyone knows that if you don't breathe well or sleep well, you won't feel well. However, despite knowing that all humans have a propensity to suffer from breathing problems while sleeping, it's rare that this information is applied at all. For example, women will tell me that they've noticed for years that their husbands stop breathing and gasp for air while sleeping, and didn't realize that it was major problem. Children who snore heavily are routinely placed on stimulant medications. Physicians, despite knowing that an older, snoring man with high blood pressure and heart disease is at risk for having OSA, almost never consider this diagnosis. Despite all the tomes of research into the causes of high blood pressure, diabetes, depression, anxiety, obesity, and many other conditions, the link between sleep apnea and these conditions is rarely made. Worse yet, milder forms of sleep breathing problems get dismissed until later when it's developed into a serious full-blown condition like OSA.

Whenever I see patients already diagnosed with CFS, fibromyalgia, mononucleosis, or anxiety, I find that some patients are very resistant to consider the possibility that their symptoms may have an alternative explanation. Many of these illnesses have diagnostic "tests" that support the condition. But having a positive test result doesn't necessarily exclude the co-existence of a sleep-breathing problem. Even if the sleep-breathing process doesn't cause these conditions, it can definitely aggravate them.

The sleep-breathing paradigm has profound implications when it comes to common conditions such as a simple cold or the flu, or controversial conditions such as mononucleosis and Lyme disease. Why do some people who suffer from any of these conditions breeze through without any problems, whereas others suffer for weeks or months? A perfect application of the sleep-breathing paradigm can be seen with mononucleosis: The Epstein-Barr virus is a common virus that's been implicated in mononucleosis. One of the hallmarks of this condition is enlarged tonsils. Since your tonsils are made of lymphoid tissue, like the glands in your neck, they will swell up if infected. If you have large tonsils to begin with and they get even bigger due to this infection, then your throat will occlude more easily and start the self-perpetuating vicious cycle that's been described in this book. If you have small to no tonsils, then the infection may seem like a routine cold to you. Notice that typical mononucleosis occurs in teens and young adults, when the voice box is more fully descended and when tonsils are more likely to be persistently enlarged.

The same concept can be applied to Lyme disease, allergies or a simple cold. Anything that causes inflammation which worsens an already narrowed airway can sometimes aggravate a self-perpetuating process, leading to further obstruction. If weight gain eventually occurs as a result of inefficient sleep, then it only aggravates the problem even further.

I don't want this sleep-breathing paradigm to be seen as another "condition" or "disease." Instead, based on concepts presented so far, by definition, all humans are on this sleep-breathing continuum, and so all people are susceptible at some point in their lives to various degrees. You could even say that this is a normal part of aging. In other words, the rate at which a person "ages" could be related to the rate at which a person's upper airway narrows. The routine medical conditions that we see and take for granted may be an expected manifestation of a gradually narrowing upper airway. One thing I've noticed is that people in their 60s and 70s with common medical problems such as high blood pressure or depression have a very narrow throat space behind the tongue, whereas healthy, vibrant and active seniors have wide open jaws with no crowding of the soft tissue structures.

If you are able to achieve quality efficient sleep, all your respective organs and other body parts will receive adequate blood supply appropriate for routine functioning. But when stressed due to a sleep-breathing problem, certain organs or body parts will be preferentially deprived of nutrients and oxygen. These areas include the digestive system, the reproductive system, and other end-organs or body parts such as the extremities or the skin. Add to this the hormonal and inflammatory factors that are involved, and you can see what begins to look like what we describe as aging.

Another fascinating implication of the sleep-breathing paradigm is when we consider the physiologic stress response and its effects on the involuntary nervous system, resulting in altered blood flow or hypersensitivity of the nerve endings in certain parts of the body. Notice that there are many instances throughout the book where migraine was mentioned. If it's true that most cases of sinus pain is from a migraine attack of the sinuses, then the same can be applied to the Eustachian tubes (pressure and pain) and the inner ear nerve endings (tinnitus, hyperacusis), as well as the intestines (IBS), and hands (Raynaud's). We can then broaden the definition of a migraine process to include any part of the body that has nerve endings, which is basically everywhere.

This explains why with migraines, tinnitus, IBS, menopause or Raynaud's, breathing exercises, yoga, meditation or any other form of stress reduction or relaxation helps to various degrees, but never cures the problem completely.

The bottom line is that if the problems I described in this book are mainly from a structural or anatomic narrowing, then conservative treatments will only do so much. All the cough medications, expectorants, nutritional supplements, herbal remedies, antibiotics or allergy medications can do is to improve that slight degree of inflammation and swelling, but never really address the problem at hand. With more and more studies questioning effectiveness of over-the-counter cold remedies, and with a good chance that the problem will go away on its own anyway, it's hard to know if any of these medications help at all. When you do feel dramatically better after taking certain antibiotics, as I explained previously, there may be an alternative explanation for your improvement, besides the anti–bacterial properties of the medication.

Regardless, I strongly recommend trying and exhausting all conservative measures first before attempting more aggressive options like surgery. For some people, conservative options like not eating late or changing sleep positions can produce dramatic results. Ultimately, if you want maximum results, you'll need to physically change your anatomy, whether by more conservative means (weight loss, allergy treatment, etc.) or by surgical intervention. At least, we should pay more attention to children's dental health, making sure to prevent narrowing of developing jaw structures.

Many conditions and circumstances can potentially narrow the upper airway and self-perpetuate more obstruction and arousals (such as from allergies, infections, acid reflux, stress or being forced to sleep on your back). Therefore it makes sense to do everything possible to avoid this situation. If your nose is stuffy, you now have a compelling reason to take measures to breathe better. Knowing that eating late can aggravate poor sleep and weight gain, you may think twice about having that late night snack. Not sleeping on your back is another.

There's a popular fable about five blind men who attempt to describe an elephant, but only are able describe the part of the elephant they are each touching. A man that is feeling the trunk will describe it differently from another describing the leg. By no means does this book describe the entire elephant, but maybe it is able to describe the trunk that is attached to the head, that's attached to the neck, etc. What surprised me most when I first discovered the concept for this book was how almost every medical and mental health condition seems to be linked in one way or another.

Some of the most influential thinkers in health and medicine today promote the idea that the human body is a complicated, interconnected organism that integrates the entire body with the mind. You can't properly treat one organ or area of the body without treating the whole person. For example, you can't treat someone with a sinus infection without addressing other factors such as social habits, diet, and stresses in life. Even if it gets better with decongestants or antibiotics, it will usually come back at some point in time. Conversely, you can't adequately treat depression without addressing medical issues such as allergies, sleep-breathing issues, or even weight gain.

The paradigm also has enormous public health implications. Should we all be sleeping on our stomachs on massage tables with holes to accommodate our faces? Do we need to radically re-engineer our beds so that we can comfortably sleep on our sides or stomachs? How many lives can be saved by screening for positional sleep-breathing problems before admission to the hospital? Even if only 1% of the people in this country with the various disorders I've described feel better by trying some of the recommendations in this book, think about the sheer numbers of people who can benefit, with improvements not only in quality of life, but also less sick days, and fewer doctor's office visits.

It's unrealistic to believe that entire industries will change to accommodate the concepts in this book. However, my hope is that individually, you'll find at least one to two simple tips or suggestions that will allow you to achieve more fulfilling and restful sleep. I'm confident that for some of you, it may even save your life.

There seems to be a dichotomy occurring in healthcare today. Scientific progress is advancing rapidly with stronger medicines and better surgical procedures, whereas record numbers of people are attracted to alternative and complementary forms of medicine. There are people in both camps that swear by their respective results, and others that swear it did nothing. As Western medicine becomes more specialized, along with the time and financial constraints that come along with our troubled health care system, doctors don't have time to find out about the patient's worries, concerns, lifestyle issues, sleep and eating habits, let alone the medical problems at hand. This void seems to have been filled by the alternative and complementary fields, which can often offer a more "holistic" approach. When a relationship begins to develop without any intermediaries that erode the doctor-patient relationship, healing can take place, regardless of which paradigm of medicine is used.

Now that you've finished this book, start to take action by reviewing the conservative steps described in Chapter 23. Many of the problems that we humans suffer from are a product of modern society, aggravated by poor diets, eating late, and not sleeping enough. There are many studies that state that the vast majority of the reasons for visits to medical doctor's offices these days are stress-related. You may be thinking that some of these suggestions are just common sense. Of course exercise will make you feel better. We've always been told that it's not good to eat late at night. But did anyone ever explain to you why it's not good to eat late? Why do we feel much better after losing only five pounds? The sleep-breathing paradigm provides answers to some of these questions.

Improper and inefficient breathing at night is just one of many examples that if seen from a different perspective, may begin to reveal the common branches that lead to the symptoms of disease. Hopefully, this paradigm can breathe new life into our ultimate goal of finding the true origins of health and disease.

Appendix A

Treatment Options for Snoring

I F YOU'VE TRIED THE CONSERVATIVE MEASURES mentioned in this book and wish to take care of the snoring problem more definitively, the next option is to undergo a thorough examination by an ear, nose and throat (ENT) doctor, especially one who specializes in snoring and OSA. After a comprehensive medical history and a general ENT examination, you will most likely undergo a quick and painless office procedure called a laryngoscopy, where a thin spaghetti-like flexible camera is passed through your nose in order to examine your nasal passageways, throat and voice box. After determining where potential sites of obstruction are located, you will most likely be sent for a sleep study to find out if you have OSA. In most cases, you will be sent for a formal overnight sleep study, either in a hospital setting or a free-standing facility.

Some doctors will administer a home-based sleep study. These range from a simple oxygen and heart rate sensors to a full-blown sleep study. In general, the simpler the exam, the less accurate the study. Even the full home-based studies are not as accurate or reliable as a laboratory based study. One of the main reasons for this is that, since you are attached to so many monitors and leads, if one lead comes off in the laboratory, the technician will be alerted and will come in to reconnect the lead. If this happened at home, and if that lead is an important one, then the entire night can be wasted. Hopefully, with advances in technology in the near future, this won't be an ongoing issue.

Once you undergo a sleep study and are found *not* to have significant OSA, what are your medical options? That depends on the results of your history and exam findings.

Open Up Your Nose

The first and most obvious step to examine is your nose. I described nasal anatomy and all the different reasons for nasal congestion in a prior chapter. If you have any degree of nasal congestion, that is the first thing that should be addressed. If you have nasal valve collapse, then you can try nasal dilator strips. For some people, this can make a dramatic difference. Unfortunately for many, these aids make no difference whatsoever. For others, there is a mixed response.

The next area to address is the inside of your nose. If you have allergies or a deviated nasal septum, this should be taken care of as well. One quick test to see if nasal congestion is aggravating (not causing) snoring is to use a nasal decongestant spray (oxymetazoline) for two to three nights before you go to sleep. These medications are strong nasal decongestants that should not be used for more than a few days at a time. There is the potential for addiction, but when used appropriately for short bursts, it can be a useful medication. If your snoring is much improved after using a nasal decongestant spray, then the source of your nasal congestion should be addressed. Sometimes, you can have both nasal valve collapse as well as nasal congestion due to allergies or a deviated septum. Either way, by addressing these two areas, you can quickly determine whether the nose is an aggravator factor in your snoring problem.

Other less common conditions include nasal polyps or chronic sinusitis. Some adults have enlarged adenoids, which are like tonsils but centrally located in the back of the nose. They can swell in response to allergies or infections, thus aggravating snoring.

Palatal Narrowing and Tongue Collapse

The next general area of potential narrowing and collapse is the soft palate. This is the most common source of snoring. If there is any degree of narrowing or muscle weakness in this area, and especially if your tonsils are large, this area can narrow down and collapse circumferentially. Once there is significant narrowing, the air you breathe squeaks through this narrowing, and because the soft palate has a free edge, it begins to vibrate, emitting snoring sounds.

In general, snoring treatments focus on stiffening the soft palate. The original office procedure that was introduced a few decades ago was the laser-assisted uvulo-palatoplasty or LAUP. This involves using a laser to burn and trim the free edge of the soft palate, essentially removing excess and redundant tissues. It usually has to be repeated two or three times in the office under local anesthesia. Because it's so painful, it's not performed as widely anymore, especially since the introduction of quicker, less painful options.

A subsequent procedure for snoring that was developed utilized radio-frequency energy. After administering a local anesthetic, a small needle is inserted into multiple areas of the soft palate and a small amount of thermal energy is applied, causing, in essence, a slight burn. As the wounds heal, a scar reaction occurs, leading to shrinkage and tightening of the soft palate tissue. This is not as painful, but the procedure still involves two to three applications.

Another clever way of stiffening the soft palate is to inject the scarring agent sodium tetradecyl sulfate, which is routinely used for varicose veins.[1] Ethanol can be used as well. This procedure also has to be performed two to three times for a successful outcome.

The most recent way of treating snoring is to place three small braided polyester rods inside the muscle layer of the soft palate (Pillar procedure). As the wounds heals over time, it promotes scarring and tightening of the soft palate, making it more difficult for vibration to occur, and hence diminishes snoring. The advantage here is that it only has to be performed once, and the pain is minimal compared with the laser procedure.

There are many more, less widely used procedures, but the above methods represent the major means of dealing with problem snoring. These procedures are successful in about 70–80% cases. It's hard to define success, since all the papers report success differently. The bottom line is that either you or your bed-partner must be happy with the level of snoring control. Obviously, as you age and throat tissues start to sag, it's expected that snoring may slowly return. But once a given procedure works, about two out of three people report continued silence at the one-year mark.

In my experience, there are few people who are ideal candidates for snoring procedures alone. The traditional way of screening out OSA via a formal overnight sleep study before offering a snoring procedure has one major flaw: If you stop breathing thirty times per hour with short subconscious arousals after every obstructive event, and if each episode last only for five to nine seconds, then you will be told you don't have OSA. You may then successfully undergo a snoring procedure by stiffening the palate, but still you are not sleeping well, and you remain excessively tired during the day, which impacts your job performance as well as your personal life. This can occur because most people have tongue collapse as the instigator of the snoring, causing the palate to flutter.

A few more caveats: If you have very large tonsils, and you don't have any significant tongue collapse, then removing your tonsils may be enough to cure your snoring. In children undergoing tonsillectomy with or without adenoidectomy, snoring goes away in most cases.

Although most of the snoring sounds can come from the soft palate, other areas inside the throat can vibrate as well, such as the tonsils, the walls of your throat, your tongue, and the epiglottis (a little "hood" that sits at the base of your tongue, just in front of the voice box).

Lastly, for many people, the tongue is the most common culprit. Due to various considerations discussed previously in the anatomy chapter, the human tongue can fall back for multiple reasons. If the overall volume inside your facial bones is small to begin with, then there's less room for your tongue to maneuver, making it more likely to fall back under certain conditions. In this situation, a mandibular advancement device may be a good option for you. These devices were discussed in more detail in the chapters on treating sleep-breathing problems. Notice that many of the way of treating snoring and OSA are very similar.

There are a few more interesting options that I want to mention. A number of internet programs exist that claim to help snorers, mainly via strengthening the throat and tongue muscles. There are tongue and singing exercises, and even studies that show that playing an Australian Aborigine musical instrument called the didgeridoo can help as well. All of these methods involve profound tongue and throat muscle control, presumably leading to improved muscle tone at night while sleeping. I don't think they are harmful in any way, and I continue to tell patients that they can try it, and if it works, keep doing it. I have had a number of patients that swear by some of these methods. My only concern about these programs is that it may delay diagnosis of underlying OSA.

Tips for Partners of Snorers

There are many ear plug companies that heavily promote their products for snoring, and as something that can save your marriage or relationship as well. This works sometimes, but only covers up the problem (pun intended). I get so upset whenever I see these ads, since it only delays getting to the root of the problem, and many people with OSA continue to go undiagnosed. Once I had a woman who got a piece of the ear plug stuck deep in her ear canal and it became so severely infected that it required removal under anesthesia. Obviously, not everyone who snores should undergo a formal medical evaluation and an overnight sleep study. My point here is that if your bed-partner snores, you should at least get him or her screened to make sure that there's no significant OSA. Once cleared, then you can go ahead and wear ear plugs.

One other thing that I frequently see in people using ear plugs is that they tend to push normal ear wax deeper into the ear canals. Sometimes it pushes it in so far that hearing loss results. Normally, earwax comes out naturally by itself, but whenever you push ear wax in against the grain using ear plugs or even with Q-Tips®, you're only headed for trouble. Remember the old saying, "Never place anything larger than your elbow inside your ear." It's good advice.

Although I outline in this chapter ways to deal with snoring, the bottom line is that without addressing your anatomy, your diet and lifestyle, even after your snoring is taken care of, it will most likely come back. Covering up the snoring with sleep position changes, nasal dilator strips, throat sprays or pillows only delays treating the root cause of the problem. Typically, continued poor quality sleep can lead to weight gain over many years, progressing into true OSA.

References

Chapter 1

1. Gami, A. S., Howard, D. E., Olson, E. J., & Somers, V. K. (2005). Day-night pattern of sudden death in obstructive sleep apnea. *The New England Journal of Medicine*, 352(12), 1206–1214.

2. Zanation, A. M. & Senior, B. A. (2005). The relationship between extraesophageal reflux (EER) and obstructive sleep apnea (OSA). *Sleep Medicine Reviews*, 9(6), 453–458.

3. Leggett, J. J., Johnston, B. T., Mills, M., Gamble, J., & Heaney, L. G. (2005). Prevalence of gastroesophageal reflux in difficult asthma: relationship to asthma outcome. *Chest*, 127(4), 1227–1231.

4. Loehrl, T. A. & Smith, T. L. (2004). Chronic sinusitis and gastroesophageal reflux: are they related? *Current Opinion in Otolaryngology–Head and Neck Surgery*, 12(1), 18–20.

5. Shamsuzzaman, A. S., Gersh, B. J., & Somers, V. K. (2003). Obstructive sleep apnea: implications for cardiac and vascular disease. *Journal of the American Medical Association*, 290(14), 1906–1914.

6. Schwartz, D. J., Kohler, W. C., & Karatinos, G. (2005). Symptoms of depression in individuals with obstructive sleep apnea may be amenable to treatment with continuous positive airway pressure. *Chest*, 128(3), 1304–1309.

7. Ip, M. S., Lam, B., Ng, M. M., Lam, W. K., Tsang, K. W., & Lam, K. S. (2002). Obstructive sleep apnea is independently associated with insulin resistance. *American Journal of Respiratory and Critical Care Medicine*, 165(5), 670–676.

8. Guilleminault, C., Palombini, L., Poyares, D., Takaoka, S., Huynh, N. T., & El-Sayed, Y. (2008). Pre-eclampsia and nasal CPAP: Part 1. Early intervention with nasal CPAP in pregnant women with risk factors for pre-eclampsia: preliminary findings. *Sleep Medicine*, 9(1), 9–14.

9. Poyares, D., Guilleminault, C., Hachul, H., Fujita, L., Takaoka, S., Tufik, S., & Sass, N. (2008). Pre-eclampsia and nasal CPAP: Part 2. Hypertension

during pregnancy, chronic snoring, and early nasal CPAP intervention. *Sleep Medicine,* 9(1), 15–21.

10. Aviv, J. E., Liu, H., Parides, M., Kaplan, S. T., & Close, L. G. (2000). Laryngopharyngeal sensory deficits in patients with laryngopharyngeal reflux and dysphagia. *The Annals of Otology, Rhinology, and Laryngology,* 109(11), 1000–1006.

11. Mortimore, I. L. & Douglas, N. J. (1997). Palatal muscle EMG response to negative pressure in awake sleep apneic and control subjects. *American Journal of Respiratory and Critical Care Medicine,* 156(3 Pt 1), 867–873.

Chapter 2

1. Davidson, T. M. (2003). The Great Leap Forward: the anatomic basis for the acquisition of speech and obstructive sleep apnea. *Sleep Medicine,* 4(3), 185–194.

2. Price W. J. (1945). *Nutrition and physical degeneration.* 6th ed. La Mesa: Price-Pottenger, 1945.

3. Palmer B. J. (2003). The uniqueness of the human airway (Parts I and II). *Sleep Review,* 4(2), 40–43; 4(3), 54–58.

Chapter 3

1. Young, T., Peppard, P. E., & Gottlieb, D. J. (2002). Epidemiology of obstructive sleep apnea: a population health perspective. *American Journal of Respiratory and Critical Care Medicine,* 165(9), 1217–1239.

2. Young, T., Evans, L., Finn, L., & Palta, M. (1997). Estimation of the clinically diagnosed proportion of sleep apnea syndrome in middle-aged men and women. *Sleep,* 20(9), 705–706.

3. Guilleminault, C., Stoohs, R., Clerk, A., Cetel, M., & Maistros, P. (1993). A cause of excessive daytime sleepiness. The upper airway resistance syndrome. *Chest,* 104(3), 781–787.

4. Guilleminault, C., Faul, J. L., & Stoohs, R. (2001). Sleep-disordered breathing and hypotension. *American Journal of Respiratory and Critical Care Medicine,* 164(7), 1242–1247.

5. Gold, A. R., Dipalo, F., Gold, M. S., & O'Hearn, D. (2003). The symptoms and signs of upper airway resistance syndrome: a link to the functional somatic syndromes. *Chest,* 123(1), 87–95.

Chapter 4

1. Elliott, A. R., Shea, S. A., Dijk, D. J., Wyatt, J. K., Riel, E., Neri, D. F., Zeisler, C. A., West, J. B., & Prisk, G. K. (2001). Microgravity reduces sleep-disordered breathing in humans. *American Journal of Respiratory and Critical Care Medicine*, 164(3), 478–485.

2. Roehrs, T., Hyde, M., Blaisdell, B., Greenwald, M., & Roth, T. (2006). Sleep loss and REM sleep loss are hyperalgesic. *Sleep*, 29(2), 145–151.

Chapter 6

1. Eross, E., Dodick, D., & Eross, M. (2007). The Sinus, Allergy and Migraine Study (SAMS). *Headache*, 47(2), 213–224.

Chapter 7

1. Levine, D. (September, 1999). Prone to panic. *Johns Hopkins Magazine*.

2. Youakim, J. M., Doghramji, K., & Schutte, S. L. (1998). Post-traumatic stress disorder and obstructive sleep apnea syndrome. *Psychosomatics*, 39(2), 168–171.

Chapter 8

1. Popovic, R. M. & White, D. P. (1998). Upper airway muscle activity in normal women: influence of hormonal status. *Journal of Applied Physiology*, 84(3), 1055–1062.

Chapter 9

1. *The New York Times*. To Have, Hold and Cherish, Until Bedtime. March 11, 2007.

Chapter 10

1. Chervin, R. D., Ruzicka, D. L., Giordani, B. J., Weatherly, R. A., Dillon, J. E., Hodges, E. K., Marcus, C. L., & Guire, K. E. (2006). Sleep-disordered breathing, behavior, and cognition in children before and after adenotonsillectomy. *Pediatrics*, 117(4), e769–778.

2. Gottlieb, D. J., Vezina, R. M., Chase, C., Lesko, S. M., Heeren, T. C., Weese-Mayer, D. E., Auerbach, S. H., & Corwin, M. J. (2003). Symptoms

of sleep-disordered breathing in 5-year-old children are associated with sleepiness and problem behaviors. *Pediatrics*, 112(4), 870–877.

3. Lewin, D. S., Rosen, R. C., England, S. J., & Dahl, R. E. (2002). Preliminary evidence of behavioral and cognitive sequelae of obstructive sleep apnea in children. *Sleep Medicine*, 3(1), 5–13.

4. Chervin, R. D., Dillon, J. E., Bassetti, C., Ganoczy, D. A., & Pituch, K. J. (1997). Symptoms of sleep disorders, inattention, and hyperactivity in children. *Sleep*, 20(12), 1185–1192.

5. Naseem, S., Chaudhary, B., & Collop, N. (2001). Attention deficit hyperactivity disorder in adults and obstructive sleep apnea. *Chest*, 119(1), 294–296.

Chapter 11

1. Nishizawa, T., Akaoka, I., Nishida, Y., Kawaguchi, Y., & Hayashi, E. (1976). Some factors related to obesity in the Japanese sumo wrestler. *The American Journal of Clinical Nutrition*, 29(10), 1167–1174.

Chapter 12

1. Edwards, N., Blyton, D. M., Kirjavainen, T., Kesby, G. J., & Sullivan, C. E. (2000). Nasal continuous positive airway pressure reduces sleep-induced blood pressure increments in preeclampsia. *American Journal of Respiratory and Critical Care Medicine*, 162(1), 252–257.

2. Franklin, K. A., Holmgren, P. A., Jönsson, F., Poromaa, N., Stenlund, H., & Svanborg, E. (2000). Snoring, pregnancy-induced hypertension, and growth retardation of the fetus. *Chest*, 117(1), 137–141.

3. Lee, K. A. & Gay, C. L. (2004). Sleep in late pregnancy predicts length of labor and type of delivery. *American journal of obstetrics and gynecology*, 191(6), 2041–2046.

Chapter 15

1. Lavie, L., Kraiczi, H., Hefetz, A., Ghandour, H., Perelman, A., Hedner, J., & Lavie, P. (2002). Plasma vascular endothelial growth factor in sleep apnea syndrome: effects of nasal continuous positive air pressure treatment. *American Journal of Respiratory and Critical Care Medicine*, 165(12), 1624–1628.

2. Duffy, J. P., Eibl, G., Reber, H. A., & Hines, O. J. (2003). Influence of hypoxia and neoangiogenesis on the growth of pancreatic cancer. *Molecular Cancer*, 2, 12.

3. Blagosklonny, M. V. (2001). Hypoxia-inducible factor: Achilles' heel of antiangiogenic cancer therapy (review). *International Journal of Oncology*, 19(2), 257–262.

4. Pugh, C. W. & Ratcliffe, P. J. (2003). Regulation of angiogenesis by hypoxia: role of the HIF system. *Nature Medicine*, 9(6), 677–684.

5. Fei, P., Wang, W., Kim, S. H., Wang, S., Burns, T. F., Sax, J. K, Buzzai, M., Dicker, D. T., McKenna, W. G., Bernard, E. J., & El-Deiry, W.S. (2004). Bnip3L is induced by p53 under hypoxia, and its knockdown promotes tumor growth. *Cancer Cell*, 6(6), 597–609.

6. Shamsuzzaman, A. S., Gersh, B. J., & Somers, V. K. (2003). Obstructive sleep apnea: implications for cardiac and vascular disease. *Journal of the American Medical Association*, 290(14), 1906–1914.

7. Pressman, M. R., Figueroa, W. G., Kendrick-Mohamed, J., Greenspon, L. W., & Peterson, D. D. (1996). Nocturia. A rarely recognized symptom of sleep apnea and other occult sleep disorders. *Archives of Internal Medicine*, 156(5), 545–50.

Chapter 16

1. Yaggi, H. K., Concato, J., Kernan, W. N., Lichtman, J. H., Brass, L. M., & Mohsenin, V. (2005). Obstructive sleep apnea as a risk factor for stroke and death. *The New England Journal of Medicine*, 353(19), 2034–2041.

Chapter 19

1. Wetmore, S. J., Scrima, L., & Hiller, F. C. (1988). Sleep apnea in epistaxis patients treated with nasal packs. *Otolaryngology–Head and Neck Surgery*, 98(6), 596–599.

2. DiBaise, J. K., Olusola, B. F., Huerter, J. V., & Quigley, E. M. (2002). Role of GERD in chronic resistant sinusitis: a prospective, open label, pilot trial. *The American Journal of Gastroenterology*, 97(4), 843–850.

3. Senior, B. A., Khan, M., Schwimmer, C., Rosenthal, L., & Benninger, M. (2001). Gastroesophageal reflux and obstructive sleep apnea. *The Laryngoscope*, 111(12), 2144–2146.

4. Tessema, B., Leoniak, S., & Park, SY. (2007). Obstructive sleep apnea in patients with recalcitrant chronic rhinosinusitis. Presented at the 53th Annual Meeting of the American Rhinologic Society, Washington DC, September.

Chapter 20

1. Friedman, M., Ibrahim, H., Syed, Z. (2003). Nasal valve suspension: an improved, simplified technique for nasal valve collapse. *Laryngoscope*, 113(2), 381–385.

Chapter 21

1. National Sleep Foundation (2005). Sleep In America Poll.

2. Lugaresi, E., Cirignotta, F., Coccagna, G., & Baruzzi, A. (1982). Snoring and the obstructive apnea syndrome. *Electroencephalography and Clinical Neurophysiology (Supplement)*, 35, 421–430.

3. Fairbanks, D., Mickelson, S., & Woodson, BT. (2003). *Snoring and Obstructive Sleep Apnea*. Philadelphia: Lippincott Williams & Wilkins.

4. Young, T., Evans, L., Finn, L., & Palta, M. (1997). Estimation of the clinically diagnosed proportion of sleep apnea syndrome in middle-aged men and women. *Sleep*, 20(9), 705–706.

5. Kimoff, R. J., Sforza, E., Champagne, V., Ofiara, L., & Gendron, D. (2001). Upper airway sensation in snoring and obstructive sleep apnea. *American Journal of Respiratory and Critical Care Medicine*, 164 (2), 250–255.

6. Amatoury, J., Howitt, L., Wheatley, J. R., Avolio, A. P., & Amis, T. C. (2006). Snoring-related energy transmission to the carotid artery in rabbits. *Journal of Applied Physiology*, 100(5), 1547–1553.

7. Silvestrini, M., Rizzato, B., Placidi, F., Baruffaldi, R., Bianconi, A., & Diomedi, M. (2002). Carotid artery wall thickness in patients with obstructive sleep apnea syndrome. *Stroke*, 33(7), 1782–1785.

8. Collop, N. (2007). The effect of obstructive sleep apnea on chronic medical disorders. *Cleveland Clinic Journal of Medicine*, 74(1), 72–78.

9. Peppard, P. E., Young, T., Palta, M., & Skatrud, J. (2000). Prospective study of the association between sleep-disordered breathing and hypertension. *The New England Journal of Medicine*, 342(19), 1378–1384.

10. Lewin, D. S., Rosen, R. C., England, S. J., & Dahl, R. E. (2002). Preliminary evidence of behavioral and cognitive sequelae of obstructive sleep apnea in children. *Sleep Medicine*, 3(1), 5–13.

11. Lu, L. R., Peat, J. K., & Sullivan, C. E. (2003). Snoring in preschool children: prevalence and association with nocturnal cough and asthma. *Chest*, 124(2), 587–593.

12. Michaelson, P. G. & Mair, E. A. (2004). Popular snore aids: do they work? *Otolaryngology–Head and Neck Surgery*, 130 (6), 649–658.

13. *The New York Times*. To Have, Hold and Cherish, Until Bedtime. March 11, 2007.

Chapter 23

1. Freire, A. O., Sugai, G. C., Chrispin, F. S., Togeiro, S. M., Yamamura, Y., Mello, L. E., & Tufik, S. (2007). Treatment of moderate obstructive sleep apnea syndrome with acupuncture: a randomised, placebo-controlled pilot trial. *Sleep Medicine*, 8(1), 43–50.

Chapter 25

1. Sher, A. E., Schechtman, K. B., & Piccirillo, J. F. (1996). The efficacy of surgical modifications of the upper airway in adults with obstructive sleep apnea syndrome. *Sleep*, 19(2), 156–177.

2. Weaver, E. M., Maynard, C., & Yueh, B. (2004). Survival of veterans with sleep apnea: continuous positive airway pressure versus surgery. *Otolaryngology–Head and Neck Surgery*, 130(6), 659–665.

3. Riley, R. W., Powell, N. B., & Guilleminault, C. (1993). Obstructive sleep apnea syndrome: a review of 306 consecutively treated surgical patients. *Otolaryngology–Head and Neck Surgery*, 108(2), 117–125.

4. Friedman, M., Ibrahim, H., & Joseph, N. J. (2004). Staging of obstructive sleep apnea/hypopnea syndrome: a guide to appropriate treatment. *The Laryngoscope*, 114(3), 454–459.

5. Maturo, S. C. & Mair, E. A. (2006). Submucosal minimally invasive lingual excision: an effective, novel surgery for pediatric tongue base reduction. *The Annals of Otology, Rhinology, and Laryngology*, 115(8), 624–630.

6. Riley, R. W., Powell, N. B., & Guilleminault, C. (1994). Obstructive sleep apnea and the hyoid: a revised surgical procedure. *Otolaryngology–Head and Neck Surgery*, 111(6), 717–721.

7. Jacobowitz, O. (2006). Palatal and tongue base surgery for surgical treatment of obstructive sleep apnea: a prospective study. (2006) *Otolaryngology–Head and Neck Surgery*, 135, 258–264.

8. Omur, M., Ozturan, D., Elez, F., Unver, C., & Derman, S. (2005). Tongue base suspension combined with UPPP in severe OSA patients. *Otolaryngology–Head and Neck Surgery*, 133, 218–223.

9. Vicente, E., Marin, J.M., Carrizo, S., Naya, M.J. (2006). Tongue-base suspension in conjunction with uvulopalatopharyngoplasty for treatment of severe obstructive sleep apnea: long-term follow-up results. *Laryngoscope*, 116(7), 1223–1227.

Appendix

1. Brietzke, S. E. & Mair, E. A. (2001). Injection snoreplasty: how to treat snoring without all the pain and expense. *Otolaryngology–Head and Neck Surgery*, 124(5), 503–510.

Index

acid reflux
  antibiotics for, 48
  asthma and, 5
  causes of, 6–7, 20, 38, 49
  GERD and, 5–9, 169
  H. pylori bacterium and,
    50, 52
  LPRD and, 5, 49–50, 169
  meal times and, 169
  nasal congestion and, 51–3
  OSA and, 5
  pepsin, 49–50
  throat, 49–50
  tongue collapse and, 34–6, 49
  UARS and, 5
  vacuum effect and, 6–7, 20,
    38, 49
acupuncture, stress control and,
  179
adenoidectomies
  ADHD and, 74–7

children's behavior improved
  by, 56–7
adenoids
  nasal congestion and, 143
  removal of, 56–7, 74–7, 143
  snoring and swelling of,
    216–7
"adrenal burnout syndrome," CFS
  as, 123–4
adrenocorticotropic hormone, 114
alcohol consumption, sleep quality
  and, 90, 131, 151, 158, 176
allergic rhinitis, 52
allergies
  nasal, 52, 169–72
  pet, 170–1
alpha-delta sleep, UARS and, 28
antibiotics
  azithromycin, 52
  over-prescribed, 47–8, 52
anxiety
  OSA, 57, 60–1

Guilleminault, Christian, 27–8

H. pylori bacterium, 50, 52
headaches
    deviated septum and, 53
    migraine, 28, 52–3, 96, 209–10
    sinus, 5, 51–3, 209–10
    UARS and, 28, 96
hearing loss, sudden, 129–30
heart attacks
    breathing obstructions and,
        36–8
    OSA and, 25–6, 107–11
    sleep and, 4–5
    timing of, 4–5, 36
heart disease
    napping and, 175
    OSA and, 25–6, 107–11
high blood pressure, OSA and,
    107–11
high-energy density foods, 83
hormone levels, sleep disorders
    and, 114–7
hormones. *See* hormone levels *and*
    particular hormones.
hot flashes, sleep-breathing
    conditions and, 63–7, 157
hunger, hormone levels and, 79–80,
    115–7
hyoid myotomy with suspension
    (HMS), 203–5
hyperacusis, 130
hyperthyroidism
    "adrenal burnout syndrome"
        and 123–4
    OSA and, 124
    sleep-breathing conditions
        and, 28, 115
    sleep deprivation and, 121–3
    UARS and, 28

hypocretin, 115
hypopnea, 25. *See also* apnea
    hypopnea index *and* obstructive
    sleep apnea.
hypoxia, 8, 102–4, 109, 122

immune system, sleep and health
    of, 102, 104
infertility
    sleep problems and, 71–2
    stress and, 72
insomnia
    causes of, 90–3
    countering, 179–82
    depression and, 91–2
    OSA and, 90
    sleep-breathing conditions
        and, 90–3, 157–8
    sleep-maintenance, 89–90
    sleep-onset, 28, 89–90
    sleep position and, 90–2
    types of, 89–90
    UARS and, 28, 91
involuntary nervous system, 177
irritable bowel syndrome (IBS)
    alpha-delta sleep and, 28
    sleep deprivation and, 121–3
    UARS and, 28, 97

klinorynchy, 14, 16

language acquisition,
    consequences of, 13–6
laryngeal descent, 14–5
laryngopharyngeal reflux disease
    (LPRD)
    chronic sinusitis and, 5
    conditions associated with,
        49–50

About the Author

D<small>R.</small> S<small>TEVEN</small> Y. P<small>ARK</small> sees patients in his private practice in New York City. He is a board-certified otolaryngologist with a B.A. in biophysics from The Johns Hopkins University, and his medical degree from Columbia University. Dr. Park is a clinical assistant professor of otolaryngology at the New York Medical College, and is active in teaching medical students, residents and fellows in training. He is frequently invited as a guest lecturer for various organizations and academic conferences, to share his unique insight into his sleep-breathing paradigm. For more information, you can email him at info@sleepinterrupted.com.

Quick Order Form

5 Easy Ways to Place Your Order:

Web: www.sleepinterrupted.com
Email: orders@sleepinterrupted.com
Fax: 212-315-9558 (send this form)
Telephone: 866-693-1115 toll-free (have your credit card ready)
Mail: Jodev Press, LLC. 330 W. 58th Street, Suite 610, New York, NY 10019

> ❏ Please send _____ copies of **Sleep, Interrupted** @ US $24.99 each
> (For bulk orders, please call)

Subtotal: _____

8.375% Sales tax (for books shipped to NY State): _____

Shipping (US $4 for first book and $2 for each additional book): _____
International (US $9 for first book and $5 for each additional book)

Total: _____

I understand that I may return any undamaged copies within 30 days for a full refund – for any reason, no questions asked.

Please email me more FREE information on (circle):

| Diet/nutrition | Weight loss | Chronic fatigue | Stress relief |
| Hormone issues | Sinusitis | Athletic performance | Smoking cessation |

Name: _____ Email: _____

Shipping address: _____

City: _____ State: _____ Zip: _____

Telephone: _____

Payment (circle):   Check*   Visa   MasterCard   Amex

Card number: _____ Exp.: _____

Billing address (if different from above):

Address: _____

City: _____ State: _____ Zip: _____

Comments: _____
* Please make checks payable to Jodev Press, LLC

OSA
~~OAS~~ = obstructive sleep apnea

U ARS = upper airway resistance
syndrome

L P RD = laryngopharyngeal reflux
disease

GERD = gastro esophageal reflux
disease